Healing, Hype or Harm?

A Critical Analysis of Complementary
or Alternative Medicine

Edited by
Edzard Ernst

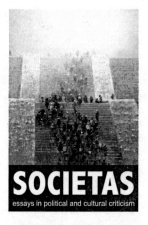

SOCIETAS
essays in political and cultural criticism

imprint-academic.com/societas

Published in the UK by Societas
Imprint Academic, PO Box 200, Exeter EX5 5YX, UK

Published in the USA by Societas
Imprint Academic, Philosophy Documentation Center
PO Box 7147, Charlottesville, VA 22906-7147, USA

ISBN 9781845401184

A CIP catalogue record for this book is available from the
British Library and US Library of Congress

Contents

Contributors

Michael Baum
The Portland Hospital
Great Portland Street
London W1N 6AH
Michael@mbaum.freeserve.co.uk

Kate Boddy
Complementary Medicine
Peninsula Medical School
25 Victoria Park Road
Exeter EX2 4NT
k.boddy@ex.ac.uk

Gustav Born
William Harvey Research Inst.
Charterhouse Square
London EC1M 6BQ
g.v.born@qmul.ac.uk

Peter H. Canter
Complementary Medicine
Peninsula Medical School
[as above, Boddy]
peter.canter@pms.ac.uk

Bruce Charlton
School of Psychology,
Newcastle University
Newcastle NE1 7RU
bruce.charlton@newcastle.ac.uk

David Colquhoun
Department of Pharmacology
University College London
Gower Street
London WC1E 6BT
d.colquhoun@ucl.ac.uk

Edzard Ernst
Complementary Medicine
Peninsula Medical School
[as above, Boddy]
Edzard.Ernst@pms.ac.uk

Michael Fitzpatrick
Barton House Health Centre
London N16 9JT
fitz@easynet.co.uk

John Garrow
Johngarrow@aol.com

Asbjørn Hróbjartsson
The Nordic Cochrane Centre
Rigshospitalet, Copenhagen
ah@cochrane.dk

Stéphane Lejeune,
stephane.lejeune@eortc.be

Terry Polevoy
938 King Street West
Kitchener, Ontario N2G 1G4
tpinfo@healtcare.net

James Randi
randi@randi.org

Leslie Rose
Pharmavision Consulting Ltd.
11 Montague Road
West Harnham
Salisbury SP2 8NJ
lesrose@ntlworld.com

Hazel Thornton
Dept of Health Sciences
University of Leicester
hazelcagct@keme.co.uk

Barbara Wider
Complementary Medicine
Peninsula Medical School
[as above, Boddy]
b.wider@exeter.ac.uk

Nick Ross

Foreword

I am a sceptic. Maybe it's inbred personality, maybe it's years of working as a journalist, but give me a fact and I will want its provenance, tell me a story and I'm your archetypal doubting Thomas. I am no scientist, but I have come to recognise that most of the great advances by humanity have developed from the systematic form of scepticism we call the scientific method, which is to say they have been based on logical trial and error. Even the greatest temples to the gods were constructed on scientific principles; if not they tended to fall down. The more systematic the measurement and testing the greater the pace of progress, with more discoveries in the past two centuries than in all the millennia that went before.

In many ways science is the antithesis of faith. Science attempts to reject dogma not indulge in it. Good science is intrinsically heretical. In fact nearly all of its most wondrous discoveries are thoroughly counterintuitive, not least that the earth is a sphere and we are not at the centre of the cosmos, that the universe evolved creating life within the seas and hoisting seashells onto mountaintops, and that if people were to fly into the heavens we had to stop flapping.

I say science is the *antithesis* of faith because there has always been a temptation to find common ground. Most of great religions could always burn or imprison those like Galileo whose iconoclasm threatened their power over the people, but they could not resist the logic of science for ever. As Isaac Asimov famously observed, reason's victory over faith became tangible when churches began installing lightening conductors. Some fundamentalists hold out, repudiating Darwin or even Copernicus and not bothering their heads with the likes of Einstein, but on the basis that if you can't beat them join them, most religions attempt to incorporate scientific concepts into their own systems of belief.

Now we see a campaign to integrate faith and science for the treatment of disease. Indeed, why should orthodox treatment not open its arms to the alternative therapists and provide a truly 'holistic' model of healing? Well, I can see the attractions. So far as alternativists are concerned it would be good to cash in on some of the status — and cash itself — which has been earned by mainstream medicine. And for doctors, most all of whom are acutely short of time to spend with patients, almost anything that relieves the pressures on them must be appealing.

Hence this book of essays which explores the implications.

For my own part I come back to my contention that faith and science are *antithetical*. Medicine is a relative newcomer to science. Until right up to the twentieth century it remained in the grip of ancient myths promoted by those early high priests of medicine, the Greek Hippocrates and the Roman Galen, and its shameful history is worth recalling. To give those two pioneers due credit they did both acquire a good deal of anatomical knowledge and Galen was a pioneering surgeon, but their very successes lent weight to some dangerous ideas. They theorised that the four seasons of the year had counterparts in four 'humours' in the human body, and that blood, yellow bile, black bile and phlegm dictated people's personalities — sanguine, choleric, melancholic or phlegmatic. Sadly, their imagination took them beyond harmless conjecture and convinced them that it was an imbalance in these four humours which caused disease. Because of their huge reputations, for generation after generation of sick and dying patients, mainstream treatment involved a great deal of bloodletting and poisonous emetics.

This primitive approach endured until the age of deference began to founder. It survived the best endeavours of William Harvey (who discovered the circulation of blood), Louis Pasteur (who discovered germs) and many like them, and it was not until after the second world war that scientific rigour began to be widely applied. The term 'evidence-based medicine' has only been meaningful for twenty years or so, and even now many medical students graduate with little comprehension of scientific methods — as I can testify from my experience with a medical charity when trying to hand out research grants to doctors who plainly do not know how to design reliable and meaningful experiments. In fact the medical establishment still talks of medicine as, 'both a science and an art' without acknowledging the distinction and without realising implicit contradictions.

By 'art', of course, they mean intuition, guesswork and gut feeling. We humans rely on that a lot. Our brains seems to be hard-wired for anecdotes, and we learn most easily through compelling stories; but

I am aghast that so many people, including quite a number of my friends, cannot see the pitfalls in this approach. Science knows that anecdotes and personal experiences can be fatally misleading. It requires results that are testable and repeatable. Medicine, on the other hand, can only take science so far. There is too much human variability to be sure about anything very much when it comes to individual patients, so yes there is often a great deal of room for hunch. But let us be clear about the boundaries, for if we stray over them the essence of science is quickly betrayed: corners get cut and facts and opinions intermingle until we find it hard to distinguish one from the other.

As a result of this confusion conventional medicine is not as scientific people tend to think. *Some* of it is: nowadays a new medicine must go through all the hoops of careful scientific protocol, but once launched—unless there are obviously serious adverse events as there were with cardiovascular problems in some patients on Vioxx—it will drop into a dark void of largely unaudited outcomes. There are sometimes attempts to achieve professional consensus based on the best scientific evidence, and in Britain the creation of NICE (the National Centre for Health & Clinical Excellence) has for the first time put treatments into an objective framework about safety and efficacy. But why, when medicine is still in the process of dragging itself onto an evidence-based platform, should it contemplate sharing its stage with a jumble of new-age pseudoscience and age-old nonsense like meridians and astrology and with people who neither understand nor respect its progressively more scientific methods? Let's face it, the 'integrative health' approach is championed by people (and princes) who are not the most scientifically literate of people, and nor do their often privileged circles take the scientific community to heart.

No doubt there is room for some accommodation. This book rightly, if untidily, has 'Complementary *or* Alternative Medicine' in the title because there is a difference. The alternativists regard scientific methods as crudely reductionist and irrelevant, which is fine by me if their patients are basically healthy — though nauseatingly dangerous if their patients are really ill. When I first met Michael Baum he showed me women who had suppurating sores because charlatans had kept them away from real clinical expertise. Complementary therapists, on the other hand, acknowledge that science has a role, albeit many of them seem to have little real grasp of what science is all about. How else could they peddle snake oil or promote medical interventions for which the evidence of efficacy is so scant?

But here's the rub. As soon as an unorthodox approach is proved to be efficacious it becomes mainstream. In fact for all the clamour about 'natural remedies' as opposed to scientific medicine, the scientific approaches are inescapably rooted in nature and many of the most successful ones are adaptations of age-old methods—setting simple fractures for example. Indeed the first and most successful modern medicine, aspirin, is essentially a distilled form of tree bark that has been used for pain relief and inflammation since antiquity. Yes, it is the distillation that makes modern medicine so powerful, and indeed sometimes so perilous, and on occasions doctors are too quick to use potent drugs instead of mild ones, and perhaps too reluctant to use herbs like St John's Wort which, as Bruce Charlton points out, can sometimes be effective. But the bigger fact remains: complementary medicine is chiefly left with the bits that haven't yet been shown to work, and some that have positively been shown *not* to work.

Nor is it always benign. The great claim of complementary medicine is that it rarely does harm. In fact, some traditional remedies, talking therapies and physical manipulations are downright dangerous, as Terry Polevoy warns.

Frankly, when they are not, their inoffensiveness is often testament to their impotence.

That is not to deny the placebo effect, though given the fact that most illnesses are naturally self-limiting I suspect we sometimes overstate the potency of faith-based procedures. But the more powerful a placebo effect the more careful we should be to use it scientifically.

Edzard Ernst, who conceived this book, is all for that. He has been vilified by some of the alternativist faithful who are aghast that he has applied rigorous science to their articles of faith, and they are upset because he has found so many of them wanting. But he is scrupulously fair and he has always been just as vocal when he finds evidence for a non-conventional therapy as when, much more often, he can find nothing in them. The existence of such a skilled, brave and forthright professor of complementary medicine is a tribute to the Peninsula Medical School and to the University of Exeter.

All the contributors to this book, are sceptics like me, but not cynics. They are keen to find cures, wherever they may be and whoever may be advancing them, and the cheaper and fewer side effects the better. But given the huge demand for health services, and the desperate reality of rationing, we need to be tougher in appraising conventional medicine, let alone the fringe stuff. Pseudomedicine, in any form, should be exposed for what it is.

Preface

This book brings together a range of diverse views on complementary or alternative medicine (CAM). The main and most obvious common denominator is that they are critical, written by people with a passion for rational healthcare for the benefit of those who are ill.

Complementary or alternative medicine is a large and complex field with ramifications into many other areas. The man (or more likely, the woman) in the street often has a surprisingly positive and uncritical attitude towards CAM. Critics might say that this is the result of being constantly bombarded with misinformation on this subject. Misinformation is always an unfortunate thing, when related to healthcare, it can cause actual harm to patients and to society.

Our book tries to look behind the various smoke screens that tend to obstruct our vision and often prevent us from understanding the truth. The authors of this volume have very different backgrounds and views but they are all well-informed critics who do not dismiss CAM lightly. If they disapprove of certain aspects, they do so for well-argued reasons.

Proponents of CAM should consider the criticism that emerges from these essays carefully — they are unlikely to agree with it but, at the very least, they will find them thought-provoking. Those who are sceptical about CAM will find much in this book that helps them broaden their view on the subject. And the many people who have an interest in CAM but do not hold strong opinions either way may find this book a refreshing contribution counterbalancing the plethora of naively uncritical books on the subject.

Criticism, I have always thought, is a good thing, particularly if it is constructive. It enables us to make progress. This is why I believe this compilation of essays is an important contribution to the increasingly important question about the value of CAM.

E. Ernst
Exeter, March 2008

Barbara Wider and Kate Boddy

What is Complementary and Alternative Medicine?

Complementary and alternative medicine — what are we talking about?

Complementary and alternative medicine (CAM) refers to a diverse array of treatment modalities and diagnostic techniques that are not presently considered part of conventional/mainstream medicine and emphasises a holistic approach towards health care. Most people have a good idea which treatments are CAM (such as acupuncture, herbal medicine, homeopathy, and manual therapies) and which are not, yet there remains some confusion about how to define CAM.

A number of terms and definitions exist (see Table 1) which mostly define CAM by what it is *not*, for example, not provided in routine health care, not taught to medical students, not scientifically proven. In the 1970s and 1980s, the term 'alternative medicine' was popular, highlighting that CAM treatment approaches are used *instead* of conventional or mainstream treatments, thus clearly separating the two. Later, the term 'complementary medicine' was deemed more appropriate; it describes treatments used *in addition* to conventional medicine, i.e. highlighting that the two systems are used in parallel. Over the years, 'complementary and alternative medicine' established itself as an umbrella term. The focus of the term shifted from mainly meaning 'outside the mainstream medical system' to describing a group of therapeutic approaches with certain similar characteristics, which are discussed below. Nowadays 'integrated' or (American) 'integrative medicine' have become buzz words claiming to comprise 'the best of both systems' by combining conventional with CAM treatments.

Table 1: Selection of currently used definitions of CAM

Definition	Source
'CAM is a group of diverse medical and health care systems, practices, and products that are not presently considered to be part of conventional medicine.'	National Center of Complementary and Alternative Medicine, USA http://nccam.nih.gov/health/whatiscam/#1
'CAM refers to a broad set of health care practices that are not part of a country's own tradition and not integrated into the dominant health care system. Other terms sometimes used to describe these health care practices include "natural medicine", "non-conventional medicine" and "holistic medicine".'	World Health Organization. Guidelines on developing consumer information on proper use of traditional, complementary and alternative medicine. (Geneva: World Health Organization, 2004, xiii.)
'Complementary medicine refers to a group of therapeutic and diagnostic disciplines that exist largely outside the institutions where conventional health care is taught and provided.'	Zollman, C. and Vickers, A., 'What is complementary medicine?' in *British Medical Journal*, 319 (1999), 693–6.
'CAM is a broad domain of healing resources that encompasses all health systems, modalities, and practices and their accompanying theories and beliefs, other than those intrinsic to the politically dominant health systems of a particular society or culture in a given historical period.'	Cochrane Collaboration, http://www.compmed.umm.edu/Cochrane/
'Complementary medicine is diagnosis, treatment and/or prevention which complements mainstream medicine by contributing to a common whole, satisfying a demand not met by orthodoxy, or diversifying the conceptual framework of medicine.'	Ernst, E., Resch, K. L., Mills, S., Hill, R., Mitchell, A., Willoughby, M., White, A., 'Complementary medicine—a definition' in *British Journal of General Practice*, 309 (1995), 107–11

Which therapies are CAM?

CAM is an increasingly popular choice and numerous surveys exist examining CAM use among particular patient populations. A recent US survey found that sixty two per cent of adults used some form of CAM within the year when the definition of CAM therapy included prayer for health reasons (Barnes, *et al.*, 2002). When prayer for health reasons was excluded from the definition, the percentage decreased to thirty six per cent. It is important, then, to know what we mean when we talk about CAM. Table 2 contains definitions of twenty of the most commonly used CAM therapies:

Table 2: Description of CAM therapies

Therapy	Description
Acupuncture	Insertion of needles into the skin at special sites, known as points, for therapeutic or preventive purposes
Alexander technique	Psychophysical re-education to improve postural balance and coordination
Applied kinesiology	Diagnostic technique using muscle strength as an indicator of illness or allergy
Aromatherapy	Use of plant essences for therapeutic purposes, usually with massage
Bach flower remedies	System that uses plant infusions to balance emotional disturbances
Chiropractic	Diagnosis, treatment and prevention of mechanical disorders of the musculoskeletal system, emphasis on manual treatments including spinal manipulation
Guided imagery	Controlled use of mental images for therapeutic purposes
Herbal medicine	Medical use of preparations made from plant material
Homeopathy	A therapeutic method, developed by Samuel Hahnemann, often using highly diluted preparations of substances whose effects when administered to healthy subjects in less diluted form correspond to the manifestations of the disorder in the unwell patient
Hypnotherapy	Induction of a trance like state to facilitate relaxation and make use of enhanced suggestibility to effect behavioural changes and treat medical conditions

Iridology	A diagnostic technique using signs and impurities found on the iris
Magnet therapy	Permanent or pulsed magnetic fields applied to head or other parts of body, often used with acupuncture
Massage	Manipulation of the soft tissues of the whole body using pressure, friction and traction
Meditation	Diverse range of techniques based on listening to the breath, repeating a mantra, focusing attention to bring about a state of calm
Osteopathy	Manipulation of soft tissues and the mobilisation/manipulation of peripheral or spinal joints
Reflexology	Manual pressure applied to specific areas of the feet (sometimes hands or ears) that are believed to correspond with other areas or organs of the body to prevent and treat illness
Relaxation	Various techniques for eliciting the 'relaxation response' of the autonomic nervous system
Spiritual healing	Channelling of 'healing' energy from a healer to a patient to treat an illness
Tai chi	System based on Chinese philosophy and martial arts using specific movements to enhance well-being
Yoga	A mind-body intervention including gentle stretching, exercises for breath control and meditation

As we can see, these therapies are extremely diverse. To help understand and group the many divergent CAM therapies, the US National Centre for Complementary and Alternative Medicine (NCCAM) has classified CAM and created five categories:

Alternative medical systems

These are complete systems of theory and practice. Examples of alternative medical systems that have developed in Western cultures include homeopathic medicine and naturopathic medicine. Examples of systems that have developed in non-Western cultures include traditional Chinese medicine and Ayurveda.

Mind-body interventions

Mind-body medicine uses a variety of techniques designed to enhance the mind's capacity to affect bodily function and symptoms. Examples include meditation, prayer, mental healing, and therapies that use creative outlets such as art, music, or dance.

Biologically-based therapies

Biologically based therapies in CAM use substances found in nature, such as herbs, foods, and vitamins. Examples include dietary supplements and herbal products.

Manipulative and body-based methods

Manipulative and body-based methods in CAM are based on manipulation and/or movement of one or more parts of the body. Some examples include chiropractic or osteopathic manipulation, and massage.

Energy therapies

Energy therapies involve the use of energy fields. Biofield therapies are intended to affect energy fields that purportedly surround and penetrate the human body. Examples include qi gong, reiki, and therapeutic touch. Bioelectromagnetic-based therapies involve the unconventional use of electromagnetic fields, such as pulsed fields or magnetic fields.

Is CAM available within the mainstream health care system?

The understanding of what precisely constitutes CAM differs considerably between countries. Due to different historical developments and traditions, certain therapies are firmly established in mainstream medicine in some countries but not others. For example, herbal medicine, hydrotherapy and massage are part of mainstream medicine in many continental European countries, while they are often classified as CAM elsewhere.

Similarly, the availability of CAM varies between countries. In the UK, it mainly depends on whether the patient's local primary care trust has a budget for CAM and on the GP's willingness to refer a patient. There are currently five NHS Homeopathic Hospitals where treatment is available on the NHS but recent cut backs by the NHS mean that two are currently threatened by closure. Although the number of hospital clinics and general practices providing access to CAM for NHS patients is increasing, overall availability remains very limited and no firm guidelines from the government exist.

Is CAM regulated?

CAM regulation is a complicated and contentious issue. Currently only osteopaths and chiropractors have achieved statutory regulation in the UK. Theoretically anybody, regardless of insurance, skills or specialist knowledge, could set themselves up as a therapist. This leaves many clients with very little recourse should they have a complaint. The UK government has been consulting on CAM regulation since 2000 but progress has been slow. The main problem is achieving unanimity between the numerous therapy-specific regulatory organisations that already exist. Reflexology, for example, has at least twelve governing bodies which need to be united in their approach towards statutory regulation (Naish, 2005).

Is any 'official' training available for CAM?

The rapid growth of CAM has been matched by an expansion in the CAM education sector. There is a great variety of training and education available with a corresponding variety of standards and levels achievable. Courses range from evening classes at the local college to BScs in specialist CAM therapies such as acupuncture or homeopathy. A recent review of CAM courses at institutions of higher education in the UK found that seventy CAM courses were offered through thirty-one institutions of higher education (Mayhew and Ernst, 2006). It also found that the entry requirements for these courses varied considerably as did the length of the courses, the costs and academic rigour.

The majority of CAM practitioners in Britain do not have higher education CAM qualifications. Instead they usually have therapy-specific diplomas from CAM examining bodies such as the International Therapists Examining Council (ITEC). When consulting a CAM practitioner it is therefore important to choose one who is a member of a recognised body, which has a code of ethics and conduct as well as a complaints and disciplinary procedure, and who holds professional liability insurance cover.

The House of Lords Select Committee on Science and Technology recommended in 2000 that medical students should be familiarised with CAM. Although CAM has begun to be offered as specialist modules by some medical schools, no standardised curriculum for medical students is available and debate continues about whether it should be offered at all. On the one hand its inclusion in medical schools could be seen as an endorsement of CAM. On the other hand ignoring CAM potentially puts patients at risk; CAM use is so prevalent that doctors need to be able to advise patients responsibly. They also need to be trained to ask patients about their CAM use to avoid serious adverse events that could occur through drug interactions.

Has CAM been proven?

An increasing number of CAM treatments are being submitted to clinical trials. Yet for many key questions, e.g. those regarding their effectiveness, safety and cost-effectiveness, the answers are fragmentary at best. The scientific basis of CAM is clearly less solid than that of mainstream medicine. To determine whether CAM works, one needs to look at specific treatments for specific conditions, e.g. 'does acupuncture work for headache?' rather than 'does acupuncture work?' There is now an emerging body of positive evidence for certain CAM treatments i.e. acupuncture for osteoarthritis of the knee, acupuncture for nausea induced by chemotherapy, black cohosh (*Actaea racemosa*) for menopausal symptoms, devil's claw (*Harpagophytum procumbens*) for musculoskeletal pain, ginkgo (*Ginkgo biloba*) for dementia, St John's wort (*Hypericum perforatum*) for mild to moderate depression, garlic (*Allium sativum*) for hypercholesterolaemia, horse chestnut (*Aesculus hippocastanum*) for chronic venous insufficiency, hypnosis for labour pain, massage for anxiety, or aromatherapy and massage in cancer palliation, etc (Ernst *et al.*, 2006). But there is also evidence that certain CAM treatments do not to work for certain conditions, e.g. acupuncture for smoking cessation or weight reduction, chelation therapy for peripheral arterial occlusive disease, chromium for overweight/obesity, or evening primrose oil for atopic eczema, etc. With many CAM treatments we do not know whether they work or not because they either have not been investigated or the trial results preclude any firm conclusions.

Is CAM scientific?

An often voiced argument is that CAM treatments cannot be tested in the same way as conventional treatments. This argument is mainly based on the claims that the research methodology used in conventional trials is unsuitable for CAM because a) it cannot assess holistic and individualised treatments, and b) it is designed to assess other endpoints than those used in CAM and cannot detect the subtle effects of CAM.

These arguments, however, are not truly convincing: why should a real treatment effect not manifest itself when tested in a properly designed trial? Trials are designed to minimise bias and error, and they use statistics because individuals react differently. Although it is difficult to test some CAM treatments, it is possible to develop appropriate trial methodologies to answer a wide range of research questions in CAM, including for example, trials of individualised homeopathic treatment. Advocates of CAM often deny the need for testing by arguing that a treatment has been used for a very long time and certainly longer than most conventional medicine. Standing the test of time is, however, not the same as standing the test of effectiveness. As history has shown, some treatments that have been employed for a long time turned out to be useless or harmful or have been replaced by newer, more effective treatments. There is no convincing reason why double standards should be introduced for CAM.

Is CAM plausible?

Some CAM treatments certainly seem to lack a sound theoretical basis and are instead based on a concept or a 'philosophy' that is unfamiliar or even seems far-fetched. Traditional acupuncture, for instance, is based on the idea that inserting needles in points along channels ('meridians') through which the life energy *qi* flows helps to restore the balance of *qi* and therefore health. Reflexology is based on the idea that our organs are represented on the soles of our feet. Yet neither the existence of meridians and qi energy nor reflex pathways between our organs and feet have been demonstrated. Homeopathy follows the concept that diluting a remedy, up to a point where no molecules of the active ingredient remain, renders a remedy more potent which is pharmacologically inconceivable.

But this does not necessarily mean that treatments associated with such concepts or philosophies are useless. There are treatments that are demonstrably working without us knowing how they work. Treatments might be based on an incorrect rationale which eventually is corrected with the advancement of our knowledge and experience. The question of plausibility may therefore be secondary to the question of effectiveness: it may be more important to know whether something works than how it works.

Is CAM natural?

CAM is often chosen as it is considered to be natural and therefore a better alternative to conventional medicine. It is true that many CAM forms are derived from natural sources or are aimed at facilitating the body's own healing response. A closer look at what often constitutes CAM, however, reveals that this is not always the case. Acupuncture, for example, involves the insertion of needles into the skin; chiropractic therapy often requires high velocity thrusts which manipulate the joints and spine. Nutritional supplements are frequently synthetically replicated and there is nothing natural about endlessly diluting remedies for homeopathic prescriptions.

When people refer to the fact that CAM is natural they are deluding themselves that they are buying into a system that is not only natural but is in keeping with nature itself. The truth about the provenance of some of 'nature's remedies' would, however, horrify those seeking to use a medicine in keeping with their lifestyle choices. Many herbal remedies are only available from scarce resources leading to over-harvesting and decimation of a particular plant. The hunting and poaching of endangered animals for traditional Chinese medicine products is well documented. The over-fishing of sharks for the now debunked shark cartilage 'cancer cure' is a further case in point.

Is CAM harmless and safe?

A common reason for using CAM is that it is considered safe, certainly safer than conventional medicines. It seems inconceivable to some that something considered natural should be harmful; 'natural and safe' seems synonymous with CAM. Even when a particular therapy's effectiveness is in doubt it is often still taken because it is believed that 'it may not work but it won't do me any harm'. Although some CAM treatments are associated with only mild and rare risks others are harmful in a number of ways.

A simple search in the electronic literature database Pubmed for herbal medicine case reports reveals just how dangerous 'natural' products can be. The four major safety concerns brought to light by this brief search were: toxicity, serious herb-drug interactions, poisoning through contamination of herbal products and patients not revealing their herb use to doctors. Of the first thirty-five selected case reports, eight reported hepatitis caused by herbal use, eight poisoning from adulterated herbal medicines, five dermatological type adverse events, three cardiac events, two renal failure, two thyrotoxicosis and two herb-drug interactions. Three of the above had fatal outcomes.

Similarly, acupuncture and chiropractic have both been associated with serious adverse events such as pneumothorax and stroke, as have lesser known interventions such as chelation therapy or colonic irrigation.

There are also more general safety issues associated with CAM as a whole. CAM can be dangerous when it causes the patient to be misdiagnosed or if it delays access to life-saving treatments. The case of the Dutch comedian Sylvia Millecam, diagnosed with breast cancer in 2000, illustrates this point. She opposed conventional medical treatment and twice sought help from CAM doctors. These doctors informed her she did not have cancer and instead treated her with various CAM therapies. A third CAM doctor again rejected the diagnosis of cancer instead diagnosing a blood disorder which he treated with homeopathy and supplements. Ms Millecam died in 2001 (Sheldon, 2006).

CAM is potentially dangerous when patients self-medicate. Browsing the shelves of any UK chemist or health store one can find a vast array of herbs, supplements and other CAM remedies. Many of these can cause serious complications when they interact with conventional drugs or other supplements. Patients often do not tell their doctors about their CAM use and doctors usually fail to ask patients about it. This lack of communication can only increase the risk.

The notion that CAM is safe and harmless can be dangerously misleading. The situation is not helped by a serious level of under-reporting of adverse events. The majority of CAM therapies are unregulated in the UK and as such no effective system is in place for recording and analysing the occurrences of adverse events.

Is (only) CAM holistic?

Holism does not refer to an actual treatment used but rather to the attitude and outlook of the practitioner. In a holistic approach, disease is seen as the result of a disturbed balance of physical, psychological, social and spiritual levels and the purpose of therapeutic intervention is to restore balance and facilitate the body's own healing response rather than target individual disease processes or stop troublesome symptoms. It is however important to point out that holism is part of any good health care practice and not restricted to complementary practitioners. A good doctor will always treat the roots of an illness rather than the symptoms; this is not a principle that is only applied in CAM. Vice versa, it could also be that in some cases complementary practitioners have a rather reductionist approach, particularly when they claim that 'their' therapy is a panacea for all illnesses.

Conclusion

Various terms and definitions have been used to describe CAM, a diverse group of treatment modalities and diagnostic techniques with certain similar characteristics. Some of the characteristics of CAM such as regulation and education are only valid within a given historical and societal context. As this context changes over time, the position of CAM within the health care system changes. After an initial divide between alternative and mainstream medicine, there is currently a mainly patient-driven movement towards integration of the two systems. Other CAM issues are, however, of timeless and fundamental importance, namely effectiveness testing and safety assessments. These are concerns that should be addressed before any questions about integration are raised, but unfortunately this is so often not the case. Many myths and misconceptions still surround CAM. Critical analysis of this subject is therefore crucial.

References

Barnes, P.M., Powell-Griner, E., McFann, K., Nahin, R.L. (2002), 'Complementary and alternative medicine use among adults: United States, 2000' in *Adv Data*, 343, 1–19.

Ernst, E., Pittler, M.H., Wider, B., Boddy, K. (2006), *The Desktop Guide to Complementary and Alternative Medicine* (Edinburgh: Elsevier/Mosby).

Mayhew, E. and Ernst, E. (2006), 'A review of courses in CAM at institutions of higher education in the UK' in *Focus Alternative Complementary Therapy*, 11, 185–8.

NCCAM, 'What is complementary and alternative medicine?' http://nccam.nih.gov/health/whatiscam, accessed 16 July 2007.

Naish, J. (2005), 'Stop therapists setting up with no qualifications' in *The Times*, 12 March 2005.

Sheldon, T. (2006), 'Dutch doctors suspended for use of complementary medicine' in *British Medical Journal*, 332, 929.

Stéphane Lejeune

Why is CAM so Popular?

Why is CAM so popular? Firstly, we should ask ourselves, 'Is CAM popular?' In order to answer this question, we have to clarify what we understand by 'popular'. First, 'popular' can refer to a topic frequently observed in daily conversation and in a variety of media such as newspapers and the internet. 'Popular' can also refer to the high frequency of CAM use by the public.

We will discuss the first aspect of 'popularity'. Obviously, CAM is popular in the media and in the conversations we may have with our colleagues, friends and relatives. Everyone has heard about CAM because a relative has told us they are using it or because a relative advised us to use CAM for fixing our own medical problem. No one can ignore the frequent references to CAM in the health or other 'well-being' sections of magazines or health-related internet websites. The advertising is frequent and can take different forms, e.g. the miraculous cure that the promoter is glad to sell or a CAM company which provides a pseudo-scientific message promising that the treatment has been duly 'scientifically' validated. A quick search using Google with 'complementary alternative medicine' as keywords can retrieve almost two million web pages. Nowadays, the recourse to CAM appears to be fashionable and is found within the current quest for a more 'natural' or more 'human' way of life than the one promoted by our modern society. We should keep in mind that the CAM phenomenon is not new but in fact began with the rise of the homeopathy at the beginning of the nineteenth century. The use of CAM should be placed within its historical context. We shall discuss the present context later but coming back to the nineteenth century, despite the important progress of medicine (physiology, bacteriology, etc.), serious and dangerous surgery, resulting in unnecessary mutilation, was frequent. In comparison, homeopathy appeared as soft and safe and therefore attractive to the public. Some have said that homeopathy should be commended for its success because it showed that the dangerous surgical interventions, as practiced almost 200 years ago, were pointless and avoidable as they were no more effective than homeopathy and its placebo effects.

We will now discuss the widespread use of CAM amongst the population. The prevalence of, for example, a disease, is the proportion of individuals presenting the disease in a population. Here we will not talk about disease but about the use of CAM as a health related behaviour. According to the media and some surveys published in scientific journals, the use of CAM by cancer patients is not anecdotal, and more than this, the prevalence of the use of CAM is increasing. A recent systematic review of the numerous surveys conducted on the prevalence of use by cancer patients concludes that it is impossible to give an accurate general picture. In fact, the results pooled by this review show a range of use by cancer patients among European countries with a median prevalence of thirty-nine per cent, a minimum of nine per cent and a maximum of seventy-eight per cent of interviewed patients who reported the use of CAM. In addition, wide ranges of prevalence of CAM use are observed across different surveys performed in the same country. According to the authors, this heterogeneity may be explained by the various methodologies used by the surveys. Therefore, the results are not comparable. Besides the prevalence data, the expenditure data provide us with an additional indication that the use of CAM is not anecdotal and represents a real market. Approximately five billion US dollars was spent on herbal products in Europe for 2003. Without a doubt, CAM is popular, although the data do not allow us to draw an accurate picture of the prevalence of CAM use.

We learnt in the previous chapter ('What is CAM?') that CAM methods are heterogeneous and the types of use (and users) are heterogeneous as well. In fact, on one hand, some people use CAM for 'cosmetic' purposes, e.g. as a food supplement in order to counteract the effects of senescence on their body, herbal teas are taken for losing weight or more prosaically, to control hangovers. On the other hand, some people use CAM for medical purposes. Cancer patients turn to CAM in order to maximise their chance of curing the disease, enhancing their quality of life by improving symptom control and the side-effects of chemotherapy.

How can we explain the paradoxical situation that both cancer patients and healthy people are using CAM? What could be the common ground between these different CAM users? I would like to put CAM use within the context of a global social phenomenon: the reaction against so called 'modernity'. We will not discuss here the complex sociological and philosophical concept of modernity. Broadly, the concept of modernity refers to the transformation of European societies from a 'traditional' type to a 'modern' one. Historically, this can be related to the rapid modernization of society initiated by the industrial revolution. The process of modernization involves the transition from isolated communities to integrated large scale societies accompanied by a standardisation of customs and ways of living. This is also associated with an increase in the mobility of people and goods, and by the increasing volume and ease of communication. People travel further and more often. Media and the telecommunication facilities become more economically accessible. Nowadays, telephones and TVs can be found in almost every home in Western Europe. The modernization process is still ongoing and some authors even talk about post-modernity. In this sense, so called globalisation can be seen as one manifestation of modernity, with its increased flow of communication around the world, the disappearance of some local cultures and the standardisation of ways of living, e.g. eating the same food, watching the same TV programmes, buying the same goods, etc.

Why has modernity such a negative meaning in people's minds? The modernisation of society brought a lot of comfort and benefit for people but it was also accompanied by adverse effects. Nobody will complain about living in a more comfortable and relatively safer environment, but the modern way of life with its mass consumption, has generated pollution, the waste of natural resources, stress generating ways of living and fear of worrisome technologies with great power of destruction such as the atomic bomb. In addition, the traditional form of society was characterised by strong collective representations that were dominated by religious values. Spirituality and superstition were at the centre of collective thinking activities and decision making processes. References to religion were omnipresent in the public sphere and people were living their life with spiritual values. Faith can give a sense to life and even to a person's daily activities. Faith and religious beliefs may also provide self-esteem since the believer may feel that he is occupying his rightful place in the universe.

Modern society, in opposition to the traditional society, is characterised by 'rational' values, e.g. economics, or science. Nowadays, the existence of transcendental components such as religious belief is scarce and people may miss those kinds of supportive feelings, which provide explanation of the 'human condition'. The modern way of life is often accompanied by the loss of strong bonds such as family bonds, in favour of relationships oriented towards individual interest like personal development, e.g. career oriented goals. This modern set of values can be felt to be contradictory, meaningless or even noxious.

Facing the adverse effects of the modern society, people as individuals or collectively organised in groups, will develop strategies to counteract the perceived noxious consequences of modernity and to reclaim their existence. Some of the values promoted by society will be questioned and sometimes rejected, e.g. presentation of economics as essential to society's development or the use of technology to solve society's problems These strategies of resistance can be found on several levels: the individual level with the search for meaning and the quest for spirituality. Atheists may search for transcendence through practising art, reading literature and poetry or studying philosophical theories. Believers may find it by seeking spiritual support from belief systems such as religion or 'new-age' systems. Spirituality is no longer the monopoly of the church but is spread through the various sources recognised by people as providing meaning. The technological progress of communication and the media have allowed easy and fast access to a tremendous number of sources of inspiration and reference. From home, we can access the website of the Dalai Lama and read his texts or we can discover the spiritual custom and beliefs of an Amazonian tribe by watching a TV documentary. The quest for spirituality has lead to the massive commercial publication of texts commenting or describing various philosophies and religions. Nowadays, it is not rare to find people who have knowledge of Buddhism having studied various pocket books that can be bought in the train station book store!

In their quest for well-being or for enhancing the quality of life, people are purchasing the numerous commercial products produced around well-being related themes. For example, organic food or electronic devices for removing the negative energy from the air which are sold in specialised shops or even in supermarkets. The use and the purchase of CAM products follows this trend, e.g. herbal preparations for balancing body energies or for relieving the stress created by modern lifestyles.

At the collective level, people can create or join groups of individuals sharing the same spiritual or lifestyle values. These groups are offering social support and psychological comfort to their members. The use of CAM can be a central component of those groups' beliefs and practice system. This can be seen, for instance, in the communities organised around anthroposophy.

What are the reasons that push people to use CAM, despite the uncertainties about CAM's therapeutic efficacy and safety? Following the arguments developed earlier, the use of CAM is viewed not only as a part of an individual or group's strategy to achieve a state of well-being but it is also a reaction against modernity and its values. In fact, the recourse to CAM is often accompanied by the rejection of scientific rationality that constitutes the foundation of modern medicine. In addition, the medical system is seen as a monopolistic and centralized institution reflecting the negative aspects of modern society — the excessive use of technology rather than human contact, the anonymity of the patient in the care system. The involvement of pharmaceutical industries as sponsors of clinical research is sometimes interpreted as proof of the corruption of the medical institution. CAM methods are presented by their proponents to be more human, less anonymous and respectful of the individual. CAM, according to proponents, offers all the aspects that modern medicine is presented as lacking.

We need to address the question of whether the medical system is meeting patients' needs. Is CAM an answer to the patients' unmet needs? What are the patients' needs, for example, when facing cancer? After the first shock that comes with the diagnosis, the patient will have to cope with all the uncertainties generated by the experience of the disease and ultimately, the patient may have to face his or her death. History repeatedly shows that humans are likely to look for miraculous or magical solutions when facing situations out of their control. Cancer patients are searching for an increase in their physical well-being, expecting to be cured, to have their symptoms controlled and a reduction of the side-effects of the cancer treatments. At a psychosocial level, patients are searching for support and hope in facing the disease and the related uncertainties. Patients present different coping strategies such as denial of reality (refusing the diagnosis), searching for support and sustaining hope from fam-

ily, friends and beliefs. In addition, the patient is looking for individualised care and a quality relationship with the clinician.

Are these needs met by the medical system? First the physical
needs: cancer treatment aims to lengthen patient's survival. Despite
improvements in treatment, taking all types of cancer together it
remains a fatal disease in fifty per cent of cases. At the same time,
cancer therapies are often accompanied by physical side-effects.
Second, the psychological needs: in addition to the possibility of
absence of empathy and/or communication skills from the clinician,
the under-staffed and under-funded health services cause time constraints, creating a situation that may be source of conflict with
patients' expectations. This may cause feelings of frustration in the
patient and their relatives and lead to the rejection of modern medicine perceived as an inhuman and ineffective institution.

In addition, the standard cancer treatment scheme itself can
potentially create a gap between the services provided by the medical institution and the patient's expectations. In fact, during the
treatment period the patient will be at the center of a dynamic created by the hospital staff. The hospitalised patient will be seen everyday by the hospital staff and it is likely that the clinician will visit the
patient for examination or at least to ask the typical question 'how do
you feel today'. It is likely that the outpatient will have to follow a
tight schedule of visits to the hospital for treatment and examination. This will be accompanied by various contacts with the hospital
staff. After the last treatment cycle, the patient will be informed that
the treatment period is over and is optimal according to the treatment guidelines. The patient has reached the end of the treatment
period as defined by medical knowledge and by the clinician's
assessment of the disease status. The patient will then be asked to
take an appointment in several months time for the follow-up visit
with the treating physician. The patient will be told that the treatment is now over and nothing can be done at the moment from the
clinical point of view and the patient has to go back to normal life
and wait and see if the cancer is cured or to wait until additional
treatment or salvage therapy can be considered.

During this period, the patient may feel lonely as they are no longer in the center of a dynamic involving treatments and frequent
contacts with hospital staff. In order to avoid waiting passively for a
possible disease relapse, the patient will look for everything that
could maximise his/ her chance to be cured. The patient will then be
tempted to try something else. If the medical institution has nothing

more to offer, the patient will look elsewhere and then may be attracted by a CAM practitioner's offers. By looking for something outside the regular framework of medicine, the patient as a health care consumer will investigate the offers and will chose which option he/ she wants to go for. By doing it, the patient will meet, not only their need for social support but will also gain additional hope of a cure. By taking this active role, the patient will feel that he/she has control of his/her life and the patient is no longer passive in front of the disease. In addition to feeling better, the patient may enhance his/her self-esteem and gain a fighting spirit. The recourse to CAM can be seen as a disease coping strategy for cancer patients, who attempt to complement or compensate for the shortcomings of the medical system.

In conclusion, CAM therapies are popular with a significant number of people using them for various reasons. In addition, the use of CAM is fashionable and well-advertised in the media. In order to understand why CAM is so popular, we have highlighted the case of modernity and individual strategies to counteract modernity's perceived adverse effects. The quest for spirituality, but also for well-being may explain the recourse to CAM whatever the indication for their use. We have addressed the more specific question: why cancer patients are using CAM methods without being assured that CAM would benefit them and not put them in increased danger. The reasons for using CAM can be found amongst patients' needs, not only for the hope of a cure but also for psychosocial support. In this context, the use of CAM can be seen as a coping strategy. If the best available treatments are offered to patients, the health service seems unable to meet all patients' needs especially the need for psychosocial support and for meaning, including spirituality. CAM practitioners seem to offer a service to patients which compensates for what the health system, due to organisational and financial constraints, is unable to provide.[1]

---

[1]   A language revision of this article was done by Kate Boddy.

Leslie B. Rose

Evidence in Healthcare

What it is, and how we get it

The deepest sin against the human mind
is to believe things without evidence.

Thomas H. Huxley (1825–1895)

But I saw it with my own eyes!

Most people attach great weight to personal experience. Our legal
system supports this, by accepting the testimony of witnesses, who
report what they saw or heard (or what they think they saw or
heard). There are clear dangers inherent in this and other commonly
held concepts regarding evidence, dangers which the established
processes by which we presently regulate health care products are
designed to avoid.

But I want to step outside health care for a bit, into the wider world
of knowledge. Organised societies, which we might call Civilisation,
probably arose about 10,000 years ago. As soon as people started to
talk to each other, they no doubt speculated about their world.
Despite the valiant efforts of what the ancients called natural philosophers, we really didn't know anything significant about how the
universe works until the seventeenth century, when the Age of
Reason began. Up to then, the universe was explained by inventing
supernatural beings. Over the last few centuries, a process developed for separating fact from fiction, and it is called science. What is
science? It has been called 'the crash testing of ideas'. The truth is
that most ideas don't survive the crash, and are discarded. It's a
tough world out there in science. The test pivots on evidence, and I'll
ask you now whether personal experience would be good enough
evidence for that sort of test. Maybe you will say that it is, if enough
people have the same experience, but by increasing the number of

observers you are moving out of *ad hoc* testing and into designing an experiment. But even with 100 observers, there will be problems. How would we choose them? How would we rule out unrelated factors that might affect their observations? How could we eliminate wishful thinking—seeing what they want to see?

I have just described some of the problems which are inherent in what the philosophers call 'inductive logic'. For example, we often draw generalised conclusions from specific experiences. The reason we tend to do this is that it's the way we normally live our lives. We make assumptions, and most of the time it works. A rather more risky version of inductive logic is when we infer causality, such as assuming that echinacea cured a cold because the symptoms stopped after taking the herb. Colds always clear up anyway. We don't know if the herb had anything to do with it.

A toolkit for knowledge

Science is the method by which we can reduce such problems, and as a consequence reduce the uncertainty surrounding a result. I will say now that we can never get rid of uncertainty altogether. We can however reduce it to such low levels that we run a negligible risk by treating a result as proven. For example, there is now so much evidence from observation and experiment in support of Darwinian evolution, that many people accept it as a fact. The people who don't, mostly do so by ignoring or distorting the evidence. I don't propose to go into detail here about all the many problems with reports based on personal experience (which we call anecdotal evidence), but I think you can see that such evidence has uncertainty at its core, whereas science constantly attempts to reduce it. It does this by using a very well-defined tool set. The tools include:

- Controls, such as comparison groups.
- Measures to reduce various sources of bias, e.g. observer bias.
- Using multiple observations.
- Getting the results checked independently.
- Peer review.
- Replication of experiments.

I will briefly explain what these mean. Readers who can remember their school science lessons will know about the first of these. Essentially, we are asking whether what we expect to see could have been caused by something other than the thing we are testing. We do this by setting up a kind of parallel experiment, which is as far as possible the same as the main experiment, with one major difference. We leave out the thing we are testing. This is important in all areas of science, but especially so in the life sciences, for two reasons. Firstly, living organisms are extremely complex, and we can't reliably predict what might happen as a result of something we do (commonly called the 'intervention'). Secondly, individuals even from the same species vary quite widely in the way they respond to change. So to determine whether we are seeing a real effect or just variation between individuals, we would need to test several individuals not one, and also to compare one group having the intervention with another group not having it. The second group is called the control, and this approach has another benefit if it is used in a certain way. Contrary to much popular opinion, scientists are generally not cold unemotional people who can only think like a computer. They can fall victim to the same failings as the rest of humanity. What if the experimenter reports a particular observation, which fits exactly his prediction? Should we believe him? Perhaps not. What if we learn that he knew which group had the intervention and which did not? Most people would quite rightly be rather suspicious. We need not accuse the experimenter of deliberate fraud (although it does happen), but we might find it hard to exclude the possibility that he thought he saw what he wanted to see.

This is why scientists often use the 'blinded' design. The experiment is set up so that nobody knows which group had the real test until codes are revealed at the end. The experimenter can't be biased in their observations if the groups appear the same in all other respects. I have explained this approach in some detail because it is quite fundamental to how we obtain scientific knowledge in general, and is not in any way a special feature of medical research. If we are testing the effect of a medicine in real people, we will not want them to be biased in what they report to their doctor either. To achieve this, we can give one group the real medicine and the control group a dummy or 'placebo'. Ideally the placebo will in all respects be indistinguishable from the real medicine, except for the lack of any active ingredients. Neither the patients nor the doctors carrying out the test will know who had which until after all the observations have been completed. Such a test is called a double blind clinical trial, and it is the most reliable way yet devised of determining whether a treatment works. It isn't perfect, and neither is it always well executed, but it can reduce uncertainty to lower levels than are achievable in any other way.

You will probably have thought already of two questions: How do we assign patients to the two groups (which we can call 'active' and 'placebo'), and how do we decide how many we want in each group? The most widely used assignment method is by random selection, using a list of random numbers, usually computer generated. This prevents the person doing the trial (the 'investigator') from assigning patients to the groups according to how well he/she thinks they will do—even unconsciously.

We now have in place the basic components of a fair test of a medicine, and we call this a randomised controlled trial (RCT). It forms the backbone of the highly complex process called drug development, which I will explain later. But I have not forgotten your second question. For most RCTs, the investigator will ask a statistician to calculate how many patients will be needed. This is called the sample size. The calculation is based on various factors, particularly how large a difference we might expect between active and placebo groups, and on how much variation we might expect in how the patients respond to treatment. As you might imagine, the more the variation, the harder it will be to detect a real effect. Usually, guidance for these factors will come from previous RCTs, or from other sources of data on patients with the disease we are studying.

You will not be surprised to learn that there are many variations on the RCT theme. For example, we might decide to compare two active treatments and not use a placebo. We might have three groups, two active and one placebo—this could help us to quantify the absolute effects of two drugs, rather than just to detect any difference between them. We might test the effect of adding one drug to another, and we could do this by treating two groups with the first drug, and then adding the second drug to one group and placebo to the other. This is commonly done in serious conditions such as cancer in which it will be unethical to give placebo alone.

Peer review

Even if we think that an RCT has been properly designed and conducted, we must still be very circumspect about the conclusions. Certain safeguards are built into science, which help to increase our confidence. Before deciding to publish results, the wise researcher will get someone else to check them. This internal review is mandatory in drug companies. If all appears well, the manuscript for a proposed publication is sent to a scientific/medical journal, whose editor sends it to external reviewers. This is called 'peer review' because the reviewers must be at a similar level of expertise to the paper's authors. Although valuable and essential, peer review has limitations; for example the reviewers are only looking at what they are sent and can't easily detect fraud. But there is another really valuable step. Can other researchers replicate the results? There have been many cases of amazing claims based on single studies (not just in medicine) which were overturned when other researchers obtained different results from doing the same experiment.

The empowered patient

If you have followed me so far, you are now equipped for your next visit to your doctor or other health professional. You will be able to ask whether the treatment they are offering you has been tested fairly, to see whether it works and how safe it is. But I need to warn you about the sort of answer you might receive. You might be told that there are one or two published RCTs that support the treatment. Would you accept that as solid enough evidence? Consider this: maybe twenty RCTs have been published on this treatment, and only one showed a positive result. You would be quite right to be suspicious, because you would think that the *overall* picture was one of lack of effect. The one positive RCT could easily be due to chance. Indeed, when RCTs are analysed statistically, we usually decide in advance on what we call a *significance level*, most often five per cent. This means that five per cent of the time the results will come out as positive by chance. If the significance level is below five per cent when we analyse the results (and the statistical calculations can show this), we consider this unlikely enough to believe the result. But what if your health care professional tells you about the one RCT that came out positive and quietly forgets the other nineteen? In fact there may well have been scores of RCTs carried out, with only a very few showing any effect. There is a way of dealing with this problem. Well in fact there are two ways that are closely related, the meta-analysis and the systematic review. I am not going to describe them in detail, but for both approaches the idea is to look at several RCTs to see whether there is consistency between them. But there are rules. You don't just mix up the data from all RCTs carried out on that particular medicine. What if some RCTs were badly designed or conducted compared with others? What if they measured different effects in different ways? Clearly it is important to make sure that the data structures are compatible, and that the design quality of the RCTs is high. Meta-analyses and systematic reviews, when carried out well, are considered the most reliable evidence, because they get over the problem of unfair selection of RCTs that happen to support what you want to say.

Building the edifice of evidence

We have shown that the RCT is the basic building block for testing whether a treatment works. Of course, at the same time as measuring efficacy, it is usual (and indeed normally essential) to measure safety. I'll look at the latter shortly, but right now I want to explain how several RCTs are used to build not only the top level of evidence by being grouped together in the analyses I have just described, but very importantly into an entire programme of research and development. Over the last thirty years or so, a structure has emerged for this, and we will look briefly at all the stages within it. I will take the example of the discovery and development of a typical drug. The process starts in the laboratory, with the synthesis of usually a very large number of chemical compounds which we expect to have some of the properties we want. This is a much more targeted process than it used to be, because we know a lot more about the systems in the body we want to influence. But we still have to test a lot of compounds in the laboratory to see which ones are promising. The best ones go through a battery of tests to see what positive and negative (i.e. toxic) effects they have, using 'test tube' methods (which we call *in vitro*) and animal experiments (which are *in vivo*). I want to emphasise that these tests are very tightly regulated by government agencies, and the current legislation prevents candidate drugs from being tested in humans unless this battery of tests is done without significant problems. There is a lot of debate about animal experiments, but it's important to understand that it is illegal to test a drug in humans without completing a programme of animal (and *in vitro*) testing. These tests are not of course infallible. They are a guide to what might happen in humans, not an absolute prediction, but they do reduce the risk.

At the time of writing, fresh in the public mind is a serious incident at a clinical trials unit in London earlier in the year. Six healthy human subjects suffered severe effects from a new drug which was being used in man for the first time. I am not going to analyse what happened, but it serves as an example of how such 'first into man' studies are undertaken, and importantly the extreme rarity of serious problems. This was what is called a 'phase I study'. Such studies almost always are carried out in healthy volunteers, not patients with the disease we want to treat, because we are primarily looking at safety and how the drug is handled by the body. The usual design is to test a range of single doses in a few volunteers, these doses having been established by extrapolation from animal studies — plus a substantial safety margin (i.e. the doses are lower than the doses used in animals *pro rata*). As you might expect, we also have a placebo group. The volunteers are very closely monitored on a hospital-type ward with immediate access to emergency facilities. If we don't detect anything suggesting a safety problem, the drug then goes on to a range of other phase I studies which seek to establish in more detail how the body handles the drug, for example how it is absorbed (if it's given by mouth), which parts of the body it might concentrate in, and how it is excreted. Roughly, only about one in twenty drugs that go into phase I ever get onto the market.

Phase II studies are conventionally split into two stages, IIa and IIb. The first of these is usually termed 'proof of concept', which means that it's the pivotal test of whether the drug works or not. These studies are modest in size, typically 100-200 patients with the disease we want to study.[1]

When you look at the package insert for a medicine, you usually see information about the range of dose levels that can be used. If our phase IIa trial shows on pre-defined criteria that the drug works, it then proceeds into a phase IIb study, in which a range of dose levels is tested in several groups of patients. If all goes well, we will be able to define the minimum dose that works, and also, most importantly, to show that the effects we want are dose-related. If they are, this is a major help to the doctor prescribing the drug, because it make effects more predictable.

So by now we know that the drug works, and what doses to use. Surely that should be enough to satisfy any doctor who wants to use

---

[1] We tend to use the words 'trial' and 'study' interchangeably, although the latter is a more general term which could include types of research which are not trials (such as surveys). 'Clinical' means in humans. 'Patient' means someone with the disease we are studying. 'Volunteer' means (usually) a healthy person, as in a phase I trial, although of course everyone who takes part in a trial does so voluntarily. Taken together, all healthy volunteers and patients are 'subjects', a term generally used by the public authorities which regulate medicines. It is used for convenience, and does not mean that the patient is subject to the investigator. In fact there is an elaborate legal and ethical system in place to protect their interests. There is also justification to use the term 'participant', implying a more active role by the patient.

it? Well, there remain several questions at this stage. Only a few hundred patients have been given the drug, and if it is marketed, possibly millions will receive it, so we need more assurance that it works in a typical population, and also that it is acceptably safe. So far the population has been much too small to get a decent idea of the side-effect profile. We now move up a gear, and set up what we call phase III trials. These are the pivotal trials on which the decision to allow the drug onto the market will be based. We are now looking at populations in the thousands, so usually several trials will be run. This has an added advantage as we will be more confident if several trials agree with each other (remember systematic reviews which we discussed earlier?).

How safe is 'safe'?

At this point I want to look more closely at side-effects. A lot of people are frightened by the long list of side-effects which appears on the package insert for a prescription drug. This information emanates mainly from phase III trials simply because they are the biggest. The reporting of problems with drugs is subject to the most rigorous control and regulation. The first rule is that the doctor doing the trial must report *any* adverse event (the term normally used), irrespective of whether the drug might have caused it. This helps to ensure that unexpected problems, such as that seen with thalidomide in the 1960s, are captured. Patients are also expected to report adverse events, either to their doctor or now directly to the regulatory authority. In the UK that is the Medicines and Healthcare products Regulatory Agency (MHRA). Pharmaceutical companies are obliged to devote enormous resources to capturing and processing adverse event reports. This goes on throughout a trial, and if a safety problem appears the trial will be stopped to protect the patients. Thus the list of side-effects in the package insert will often be quite long, because the reporting process is exhaustive. It does not mean any side-effect is necessarily common.

I should just make one important point about what we mean by safety. Nothing is one hundred per cent safe—it is a relative term. There can be no effects without side-effects. Our aim in drug development is to achieve an acceptable risk to benefit ratio. This will vary according to the seriousness of the condition we are treating. Drugs for cancer cause lots of nasty problems, but save lives. We would not accept such side-effects for a treatment for migraine.

Now I will not be surprised if you immediately think of celebrated drug safety issues which have arisen recently, such as heart problems with the arthritis drug Vioxx. I am not going to argue that the established drug development process, and its regulation, are in any way perfect. The problem with drug safety is that the less common side-effects can't easily be quantified in clinical trials, even with the large phase III trials. Let's consider the incidence of heart attacks. Maybe the drug is associated with a doubling in the number of heart attacks. But this is just a doubling in an already small number, so it's difficult to see statistically. This is why research and development continues after market entry, with further studies to refine our knowledge of efficacy (phase IV studies), and post-marketing surveillance of adverse events. In fact, safety monitoring of drugs never actually stops, and now everyone involved (including doctors, other healthcare workers, and patients) are able to report adverse events to the UK's drug regulatory authority.

Please revisit the list of scientific tools at the beginning of this essay. You will now see that they are all satisfied by the present process, imperfect as it is. Checking and review of results is carried out not just by the regulatory authority, but by several levels of control which start at the point at which the trial data are first recorded — now enforced by law in many countries. Within a development programme, many trials are carried out which must be consistent with each other. As the programme proceeds, a coherent picture emerges of what the drug is, and what it does.

Registration and beyond

This coherent picture is brought together as a product licence application. This is a huge body of information. All the laboratory and clinical trial data are summarised, both within and across studies. Summaries are written for individual studies, and overall summaries are written for particularly important aspects such as safety. But the fully detailed reports, and even the raw data, are also submitted, so that the regulatory authority's assessors can control what the summaries are saying. As well as all this rigorous controlling, the authorities also regularly control the organisations doing the work — for example drug companies, any contractors they use, and the hospitals and GP practices where the trials were carried out. Again, the process is not free of problems. You may well be thinking about the withdrawal of certain anti-inflammatory drugs such as Vioxx. The reason these problems arise is largely because of intensive post-marketing studies. The increase in risk of heart problems with Vioxx was in real terms not very large, and would have been

hard to detect twenty years ago. In addition, new information arising from clinical trials has to be updated into product licences—a
licence is not just issued and forgotten. Among the most recent
changes is that drug companies must publish their clinical trial
results, whether successful or not.

I have outlined how modern drugs are researched and developed
in order to demonstrate the sheer weight of evidence that is needed
before a drug can be marketed. Typically, we are looking at a ten
year process, with many thousands of candidates being discarded
for each one that becomes available to patients. We start with laboratory studies, in test tubes and in animals, move into healthy volunteers if things look promising, and then through trials which escalate
in scale and complexity. Unless all these trials are consistent the drug
will not obtain approval for marketing—and the vast majority of
drugs researched don't achieve that. So far I have not alluded to the
theme of this book, alternative medicine. I will finish with a stark
contrast. For years I have struggled to define alternative medicine,
but now I think I know what it is. It is a treatment which has not gone
through this process, and in which we can have very little confidence
that it works and is safe.

References and Resources

It is now, thanks to the Internet, very easy for everyone to access the
evidence for most treatments in regular use. Even if you don't have
your own computer, just visit your public library. Here are some
very useful websites, and I have added two recommended books.

Bandolier: www.jr2.ox.ac.uk/bandolier/
Clinical evidence: www.clinicalevidence.com/ceweb/index.jsp
Cochrane Library:
    www3.interscience.wiley.com/cgi-bin/mrwhome/106568753/HOME
Current controlled trials. http://www.controlled-trials.com/
Evans, I., Thornton, H., Chalmers, I. (2006), *Testing Treatments: Better Research
    for Better Healthcare* (British Library)
Greenhalgh, T. (2001), *How to Read a Paper* (BMJ Publishing Group, London)
Medicines and Healthcare products Regulatory Agency:
    mhra.gov.uk/home/idcplg?IdcService=SS_GET_PAGE&nodeId=5

Michael Fitzpatrick

Reclaiming Compassion

'It would be a tragic loss', writes Prince Charles, perhaps the most influential champion of alternative medicine in Britain, 'if traditional human caring had to move to the domain of complementary medicine, leaving orthodox medicine with just the technical management of disease' (HRH Prince Charles, 2001). Here the Prince of Wales touches on what Abraham Flexner, promoting a medical curriculum based firmly on scientific medicine in the USA some seventy-five years ago, described as 'a curious misapprehension' that 'not uncommonly arises' (Flexner, 1925). This was the view that the methods of scientific medicine were 'in conflict with the humanity which should characterise the physician in the presence of suffering'. But, as Flexner insisted, there was no contradiction between humanity and science—'precisely the opposite':

> For men are as apt to devote themselves to medical research and medical practice, because their hearts are torn, as because their curiosity has been piqued; and teachers, however intent on training students in the logic of practice, need not forget to inculcate, both by precept and example, the importance of tact and fine feeling. The art of noble behaviour is thus not inconsistent with the practice of the scientific method.

Advocates of alternative medicine claim that it offers a more compassionate mode of health care than conventional medicine, that its practitioners are more sympathetic and its practices more patient-centred. I believe that all these claims are false. Scientific medicine's claim to be more humane rests on its unparalleled record of achievement in the treatment of disease and the relief of suffering. Patients expect—and largely receive—from their doctors candid diagnoses and prognoses and treatments of proven efficacy (and verifiable risk). Alternative healers raise unrealistic expectations and provide therapies whose effectiveness (or safety) have rarely been objectively confirmed. The worst medical doctor can cure

diseases and save lives; the best alternative healer can only offer
false hopes.

One measure of the success of the alternative critique of mainstream medicine is the growing popularity of diverse alternative
modes of health care. A more important indication is the rise of 'complementary medicine', the tendency for orthodox medicine to adapt
to the alternative challenge by incorporating elements of this
approach within the mainstream. In practice, this amounts to a
retreat from scientific medicine to the pre-scientific traditions
embodied in the various alternative approaches. While this may
have some current popular appeal, the resulting weakening of medicine's scientific foundations risks compromising its capacity to make
further advances in the understanding and treatment of disease. No
doubt scientific medicine has many failings, but alternative medicine offers no way forward in resolving them.

In praise of biomedicine

Biomedicine stands accused of a cold, rational and instrumental
approach, of regarding the human body as a complex machine and
illness as a manifestation of mechanical dysfunction to be treated
with drugs or surgery or by some other form of technological fix.
Doctors are criticised for focusing on the diseased tissue or organ, to
the neglect of the person within which it is located, and of the wider
personal and social factors that influence the experience of illness.
Yet, if we take a historical perspective, scientific medicine can claim
that by treating the body as an object, it has achieved tremendous
successes in relieving the suffering of its human subject.

Scientific medicine is one of the outstanding products of the eighteenth century Enlightenment and it advanced in parallel with its
wider agenda of liberty, equality and democracy. In common with
modern society, modern medicine assumes the ascendancy of an
individual for whom the public world of social and political life
takes priority in terms of both personal development and in terms of
the vitality of society. By contrast, the private sphere of domestic and
personal life, in which the individual's bodily needs are satisfied,
has always been regarded as of secondary importance, both to the
individual and to society. The modern self looks outwards towards
the achievements of human civilisation rather than inwards to the
animal requirements of the human body. 'This muddy vesture of

decay', as Shakespeare puts it, 'doth grossly close' in the aspirations of the human spirit.[1]

The distinctive feature of the human condition (by contrast with other forms of organic life) is that it combines both natural and social elements. Like all animals, human beings have bodies that are subject to genetic disorders and environmental hazards, but unlike animals we also have minds that are capable of reflection and conscious intervention in society and in nature — and, to a degree, in the workings of our own bodies. For modern man, health is the default state of the human body: the absence of disease is the presupposition of active engagement in society. Illness reminds us of the unity of the body and the mind, which is ultimately confirmed by death. Shakespeare again: 'we are not ourselves when nature, being oppress'd, commands the mind to suffer with the body'.[2] Disease first diminishes us, reduces us from active citizens to passive patients, pushes us out of the worlds of work and social interaction back into the home and the sick room and, in the end, reduces us to dust. For all our creative capacities and our ambitions towards immortality, we are constrained by our flesh and blood.

Over the past 300 years the application of the methods of natural science to studying the function (and malfunction) of the human body has proved extraordinarily fruitful. Through the dissection of corpses and the vivisection of animals, through systematic observation and examination, through laboratory and clinical experimentation, medical science has developed an increasingly profound understanding of the functioning of the human body in anatomical, physiological and biochemical terms. The doctrine of specific aetiology, the notion that specific diseases have specific causes that result in pathological processes that can be identified at a cellular level, paved the way for the emergence, for the first time in human history, of effective therapies. As medical diagnoses acquired an increasingly depersonalised character, doctors came to respond to their patients' complaints in a less sentimental and more rational manner. If medical intervention in the body required professional detachment — in the case of surgery, necessitating even a degree of ruthlessness — then medical practice inevitably entailed a certain emotional distance between doctor and patient.

---

[1]   William Shakespeare, *The Merchant of Venice*, IV, iv.
[2]   William Shakespeare, *King Lear*, II, iv.

The achievements of modern medicine

According to historian David Wootton, medicine's positive contribution to humanity can be dated from Joseph Lister's first antiseptic
operation in 1865 (Wootton, 2006). In the 2500 previous years of
medical practice in the Hippocratic tradition, with their bleeding,
purging and vomiting, doctors were more likely to do harm than
good. While Wootton is highly critical of the role of the medical profession in delaying the progress of medical science, he recognises the
contribution of modern medicine to increased life expectancy in
Western society in the twentieth century. Citing John Bunker's
important study, he suggests that two of the twenty-three years
increase in longevity between 1900 and 1950 were attributable to
medicine, and three of the seven years increase between 1950 and
2000 (Bunker, 2001). He concludes that modern medicine has contributed less than twenty per cent of the overall twentieth century
increase in life expectancy (five out of thirty years), 'not nearly as
much as most of us believe' and 'much less' than the benefits of
improved nutrition and sanitation. After emphasising 2, 500 years of
failure, this seems a somewhat grudging acknowledgement of the
dramatic scale of the recent reversal in the role of medicine in society.
Not only did bad medicine turn good in the twentieth century, it got
better all the time: whereas medicine contributed less than ten per
cent of the longer life expectancy in the first half of the century, in the
second half it accounted for more than forty per cent of the increase.

Numerous medical writers have offered personal selections of
what they consider the greatest achievements of modern medicine
(Friedman and Friedland, 2000; LeFanu, 1999). Most lists include
immunisation against infectious diseases, antibiotics and the
advances in surgery made possible by anti-septic techniques and
anaesthetics. Over the past century, these interventions have saved
millions of lives and have helped towards a drastic reduction in
infant mortality and a dramatic increase in life expectancy. But medical progress is not merely measured in mortality statistics—and nor
is it confined to ancient history. Even in the thirty years since I qualified as a doctor, in a period generally regarded as one in which the
pace of medical innovation slowed, there have been many significant developments. Since the days when I worked in hospitals,
many specialities have been transformed by fibre-optics, now
widely used in diagnosis and treatment. Improved imaging techniques, using ultrasound, CT, MRI and other scans, have allowed
more accurate diagnosis, facilitating appropriate treatment (and,

scarcely less importantly, reducing diagnostic error and inappropriate treatments). When I walked the labour wards, there were no ultrasound scans, little prospect of antenatal diagnosis of congenital anomalies, few epidurals and the first IVF baby was still a toddler (she is now a mother and more than one million test-tube babies have been born). Even in general practice, new drugs have brought significant benefits. Greatly improved treatments for raised blood pressure and serum cholesterol have reduced the risk of strokes and heart attacks in older people. Effective acid blockers have virtually eliminated surgical treatments for peptic ulcers, still commonplace when I was a medical student. And Viagra has made many old men happy.

For geriatric physician Raymond Tallis, modern medicine is a 'victory of civilisation', 'over the inhumanity of the human body' (Tallis, 2004). Far from being inhumane, medical science has allowed doctors to triumph over the dehumanising effects of diverse disease processes, from infectious diseases to cancers, thereby freeing patients from the tyranny of illness and enabling them to live fuller as well as longer lives. In recent generations, for the first time in history, parents can expect all their children to survive infancy, mothers can expect to survive childbirth, and most people can expect to live in reasonably good health to a ripe old age. For this liberation from suffering on an epic scale, modern medicine deserves much credit, though even more goes to wider improvements in social conditions.

For Tallis, modern medicine is a victory of civilisation in another respect too: it is a victory over man's inhumanity to man. He cites the improvement in the treatment of people with epilepsy, once stigmatised and ill-treated, now provided with medical and nursing care. More recent examples are the transfer of thousands of people with severe mental illness from coercive institutional care into community facilities and the provision of hospice—and community care for people with terminal illness.

Condemning orthodox medicine for its mechanistic and reductionist approach, alternative practitioners proclaim a 'holistic' approach, which takes account of the patient's body, mind, and spirit. Alternative therapists regard disease as a disturbance of the harmony between the individual, nature and the cosmos; their treatment aims to assist the purposeful attempts of the body to restore its natural balance. If the fundamental principles of the alternative health movement sound familiar, this is because they are the same as those of the Hippocratic tradition which dominated orthodox medicine from antiquity until the nineteenth century (a period in which, as we have seen, almost all treatments were useless, if not dangerous). Alternative health schools claim three sources of wisdom. Some are based on revelation, either divine or secular. Others rely on speculation, theorising human health and disease in terms of elements or humours, or energy flows. Others still use empirical methods, observing patients and classifying the clinical features of disease.

Though empiricism proved the most productive approach, the activities of pre-scientific doctors were constrained by the speculative theories that guided their selection of data. As Louis Pasteur observed, 'without theory, practice is but a routine born of habit. Theory alone can bring forth and develop the spirit of invention' (Dubos, 1960). Scientific medicine emerged out of the empiricist tradition, but crucially advanced through the methods of induction and experimentation, developing theory by arguing from the particular to the general, elaborating hypotheses and testing them in practice.

Traditional healers turn ancient insights into laws of nature with eternal validity. For scientific medicine, what was previously thought to be true has often been superseded by new discoveries. Whereas traditional healers express humility in the face of nature and deference towards authority, practitioners of scientific medicine are sceptical and insubordinate, challenging divine and secular authority, questioning the evidence of the senses and the passive reflections of the human mind. 'Why think?', surgeon John Hunter famous challenged GP Edward Jenner, 'why not try the experiment?' (Moore, 2005). The historic innovation of scientific medicine was that it was open to critical evaluation and revision. Whereas alternative systems arrive in the world fully formed, medical science is in a constant state of flux.

Just as reason cannot be reconciled with irrationality, so orthodox medicine cannot be integrated with alternative medicine. For Bruce Charlton, 'fringe therapies are a kind of cultural fossil, preserving a pre-scientific and pre-critical mode of reasoning about medicine' (Charlton, 1992). Furthermore, 'their survival depends upon either ignorance or double-think (a deliberate bracketing off of skepticism) — which explains why such practices can never be disproved'. This is why the project of subjecting alternative therapies to randomized controlled trials and other scientific methods is doomed.

Just as the liberal and democratic impulses unleashed by the Enlightenment have provoked a consistently hostile reaction, so rationality in science, above all in medicine, has advanced in the face of relentless resistance. In the early nineteenth century this was linked to a Romantic sensibility, later it was associated with radical disenchantment with all aspects of bourgeois society. In the closing decades of the twentieth century, growing disillusionment with the concept of progress across the political spectrum led to a convergence of traditional conservatives and post-modernist cynics in a common suspicion of the legacy of Enlightenment rationality in both politics and science. In this climate, it was not surprising that mystical conceptions of nature, the cosmos and personal spirituality — and cults of alternative health — became more influential. The common feature of contemporary anti-humanisms is their 'devotion to primality', their emphasis on immediate thoughts, feelings, sensations and their neglect of reflection, theory, the development of ideas (Bookchin, 1995). Anti-humanists collapse the dialectical interactions between humanity and the natural world, between the individual and society, into unmediated unities: from their perspective, humans are at one with nature and with one another.

Alternative therapists reject the dualistic conception of mind and body that was first expounded by the French philosopher Rene Descartes in the seventeenth century. According to alternative health guru Deepak Chopra, 'the body is not a mindless machine; the body and mind are one'(Chopra, 1997). New age therapist Candace Pert, formerly a neuroscientist, has embraced what she characterises as the 'new paradigm', favouring the term 'bodymind' to express the way that 'the brain is integrated into the body at a molecular level' (Pert, 1997). For Pert, the 'bodymind' is part of the 'unity of life' resulting from the ubiquitous polypeptides that act as transmitters in all forms of animal life: 'humans share a common heritage, the molecules of emotion with the most modest of microscopic creatures'.

But what is achieved by replacing Descartes's mechanically opposed mind and body with a metaphysically (and terminologically) unified bodymind? The central problem, which is to discover the mediations between mind and body, is effaced by proclaiming a vacuous holism. Whereas Descartes's mechanistic approach was a historic innovation which provided the basis for modern medical science, the concept of 'bodymind' marks a retreat from science into mysticism. Pert's notion of the 'mobile brain' — what she characterises as 'an apt description of the pyschosomatic network through which intelligent information travels from one system to another' — recalls the nineteenth century notion of the mobile uterus, which was believed to travel around the female body producing hysterical symptoms.

In defence of the medical profession

The alternative critique of biomedicine is reinforced by a caricature of the orthodox medical practitioner as aloof, arrogant and authoritarian. This image has been sustained by a series of high profile scandals in the UK and provides legitimation for new modes of medical education and training and for the reform of the system of professional regulation. The bogey of the gruff paternalistic doctor offers a convenient contrast to the more feminine, informal and egalitarian style of the alternative therapist and the new wave GP alike. The most obvious defect of this popular caricature is that it is several decades out of date. The characteristic features of the doctors of the new millennium are their diffidence and defensiveness, reflecting a wider loss of professional confidence.

The more serious consequence of the growing influence of a disparaging caricature of the medical profession is that this weakens doctors' authority and undermines their capacity to relieve the suffering of their patients. In the latter decades of the twentieth century, relations between patients and doctors reflected the prestige achieved by scientific medicine in a period of sustained economic growth and social progress. Patients readily submitted to medical authority, consenting with little formality to surgery or drug treatment, temporarily sacrificing a degree of personal autonomy in the hope of alleviating their symptoms. In terms of what has been called the Cartesian contract, patients accepted a measure of objectification of their bodies in expectation of restoring their subjective capacities. Disease was regarded as an exceptional disturbance of customary good health; illness was a transient state (justifying the brief suspension of public responsibilities). The doctor had a duty to treat the patient; the patient in turn was expected to follow doctor's orders.

The current predicament of patients and doctors results from the collapse, over the past couple of decades, of the wider framework of social relations that came into being over the previous three centuries. A number of trends — the ever deeper penetration of market forces, the accelerated fragmentation of communal and family life, the decline of collective engagement and political affiliation — have gravely weakened the public sphere and have intensified individuation and a sense of personal vulnerability to wide range of environmental risks. Though the private sphere has been elevated, it has also become more problematic. The home is no longer a refuge from the world but a place of danger, from intimate relationships which are as likely to be abusive and exploitative as creative or supportive.

If the modernist self was outward looking and optimistic, the post-modernist self is depressed and preoccupied with the body (Bowler, 2004). Health is no longer a default status, but an ideal state that can only be attained through the evasion of risks and the pursuit of virtuous behaviours. This reflects the shift in the locus of disease from the body to society, from pathological cells to deviant lifestyles (though, despite more than half a century of intensive research, smoking remains the only significant lifestyle factor strongly identified with disease) (Fitzpatrick, 2004).

Making health the goal of human endeavour fosters two forms of ill-health on a large scale. The 'worried well' are people whose lives are subordinated to the quest for health, by pursuing diets, exercise regimes, taking vitamins and supplements, seeking screening tests. The 'worried sick' are those whose existential distress is manifested in physical symptoms for which medical science can find no explanation. When such patients present their complaints to mainstream medicine, they are either offered a statement that they do not appear to be suffering from any identifiable disease or they are provided with a recently coined disease label (such as ME/chronic fatigue syndrome, fibromyalgia, post-traumatic stress disorder). Neither approach offers any opening towards effective treatment. Some patients in this situation cling fiercely to disease labels which help to legitimize their distress and disability. It is ironic that while doctors try to persuade them of the likely 'biopsychosocial' determinants of their condition, some patients retreat into a dogmatic dualism, insisting on both biological aetiologies and treatments (Fitzpatrick, 2002). Not surprisingly, the worried sick provide many of the clients of alternative practitioners.

The same climate of insecurity that has led to the inflation of illness has also resulted in a loss of trust in established sources of authority, in science and medicine as well as in politics and other spheres of public life. The decline in deference to medical authority and expertise has had a number of consequences for patients. One is the emergence of the concept of the 'expert patient', which implicitly transfers a weight of responsibility from doctor to patient (Dowler, 2005). In practice, few patients are in a position to become 'expert patients', if only because of limitations of time and energy, or simply because they are ill. Campaigners against medical paternalism believe that it is patronising to suggest that doctors may know more about a patient's condition than the patient. But this is as absurd as the notion that any patient can readily acquire the information required to make important medical decisions by spending a few hours surfing the internet. While it is disparaging to medicine to suggest that expert knowledge and skills can be so readily acquired, patients are the real losers as the suffering resulting from illness is compounded by the burdens of caring for themselves.

One of the most ironic consequences of the humbling of the medical profession is that some patients have replaced deference to scientific medical practitioners with deference to alternative practitioners. Apart from the questionable theoretical basis of their practices, many alternative practitioners have not undergone systematic training and often have no effective system of professional regulation. Whereas doctors' qualifications are a matter of public record, and the basis of their treatment recommendations can be independently verified by reference to books and the internet, such protections are weak or non-existent for patients of alternative therapists. When medical doctors first acquired effective treatments, their traditional 'physicianly' bedside skills were often allowed to lapse (in the case of surgeons, even basic civilities were sometimes abandoned). As alternative therapists still have no effective treatments, they are obliged to cultivate charismatic communication skills. These may provide comfort for patients in distress; they may also be deployed by quacks and charlatans who exploit the vulnerable. It is also ironic that patients who reject orthodox doctors as paternalistic resort to alternative practitioners whose appeal is largely based on personal charisma and the authority of ancient texts. The holistic emphasis of alternative approaches, implicating lifestyle factors in both the cause and treatment of illness, is often more moralistic and punitive than conventional medicine, which in its strictly dualistic forms largely eschewed moralism (Fitzpatrick, 2006).

'What type of weapon is reason against the imperfectly understood?' — asked Michael Gearin-Tosh the Oxford don who rejected conventional treatment for his bone cancer in favour of an alternative therapy based on coffee enemas and fruit juices — and survived for ten years (Gearin-Tosh, 2002). The answer is that, in dealing with the suffering arising from disease, reason, despite all its limitations, is the best weapon we've got.

References

Bookchin, M. (1995), *Re-enchanting Humanity: A Defence of the Human Spirit Against Anti-Humanism, Misanthropy, Mysticism and Primitivism* (Continuun, London)

Bowler, S. (2004), 'Health in a sick society', Spiked-online, 3 December 2004, http://www.spiked-online.com/index.php?/site/article/1825/

Bowler, S. (2005), 'Who wants to be an Expert Patient?', Spiked-online, 31 March 2005, http://www.spiked-online.com/index.php?/site/article/1163/

Bunker, J. (2001), *Medicine Matters After All* (Nuffield Trust/Stanionery Office, London).

Charlton, B. (1992), 'Philosophy of medicine: alternative or scientific', in *Journal of the Royal Society of Medicine*, 85, 436–8.

Chopra, D. (1997), Foreword to Candace Pert, *Molecules of Emotion*.

Dubos, R. (1960), *Louis Pasteur: Free Lance of Science* (Da Capo, New York).

Fitzpatrick, M. (2002), 'Myalgic Encephalomyelitis—the dangers of Cartesian Fundamentalism', *British Journal of General Practice*, 52, 432–433.

Fitzpatrick, M. (2004), *The Tyranny of Health: Doctors and the Regulation of Lifestyle* (Routledge, London).

Fitzpatrick, M. (2006), 'The dangers of the crusade against cancer', Spiked-online, 17 January 2006, http://www.spikedonline.com/index.php?/search/results/52175752c45936542a434a30e35013cd/

Flexner, A. (1925), *Medical Education* (New York: Macmillan).

Friedman, M. and Freidland, G.W. (2000), *Medicine's Ten Greatest Discoveries* (Yale: Nota Bene)

Gearin-Tosh, M. (2002), *Living Proof* (Scribner, London).

HRH Prince Charles (2001), 'The best of both worlds', *British Medical Journal*, 322 ,181.

LeFanu, J. (1999), *The Rise and Fall of Modern Medicine* (Little Brown, London).

Moore, W. (2005), *Knife Man: Blood, Body-Snatching and the Birth of Modern Surgery* (Bantam, London).

Pert, C. (1997), *Molecules of Emotion* (Pocket Books, New York).

Tallis, R. (2004), *Hippocratic Oaths: Medicine and Its Discontents* (Atlantic, London).

Wootton, D. (2006), *Bad Medicine: Doctors Doing Harm Since Hippocrates* (OUP, Oxford).

David Colquhoun

Alternative Medicine in UK Universities

Poppleton University made history when it decided to re-name its Department of Physics and Astronomy as the Department of Evidence-based Physics. This restructuring became necessary after the foundation of the new Department of Alternative Physics and Astrology. How did this come about? The Finance and Public Relations departments at Poppleton, with rare foresight, had spotted an opportunity to get bums on seats. The old fashioned Physics Department, with its tedious insistence on evidence and mathematics, was proving to be too much like hard work to appeal to undergraduates. In the new Department of Alternative Physics, all theories are treated as equally true if someone cares to believe passionately in them, and mathematics is replaced by intuition and ancient wisdom. Consequently failure was impossible and the finances of the university were transformed. There was no problem in getting official accreditation for the new department, because naturally the accreditation was carried out by appropriate experts in alternative physics and astrology.

Of course some old-fashioned physicists deplored the fact that the new department felt unconstrained by Newton's Laws of Motion, and worried themselves about the way that their colleagues used the word 'energy' in a way that had no perceptible relationship with the way it used to be used by physicists. These curmudgeons even went so far as to complain about the university's new approach in public. Luckily for Poppleton, their complaints didn't get far. The Department of Education and the Prime Minister gave strong support to the university's 'forward-looking diversification into an emergent and non-elitist area with great revenue-generating potential' and the royal family discretely signified their approval.

The Quality Assurance Agency report was perfect (fortunately for Poppleton, they take no account of whether what is taught is true, but only about the amount of paperwork that is generated. The QAA employed that most distinguished of astrologers Russell Grant to chair the assessors, so their report could not be disputed.

The curmudgeons were summoned to the office of the vice-chancellor, who, perceiving that the university's income (and his own knighthood) were *in danger, informed them that the old-fashioned physics department would be closed altogether. The new department went from strength to strength, despite the fact that evidence for the success of its moon-lander was a bit thin. In private it was admitted that they may have failed to dilute sufficiently the rocket fuel with water, and there may have been an unfortunate error in the calculation of planetary alignments by the new sub-department of Astrology (it seems that herbal tea had been spilled over their astrolabe).*

(With apologies to the inimitable Laurie Taylor, creator of the University of Poppleton.)

Absurd? Not at all. This is precisely what has happened in medical sciences in several universities in the UK (and in far more in the USA). We haven't (yet) got any departments of Alternative Physics but we certainly have departments of Complementary and Alternative Medicine (CAM). Well, usually they call themselves 'Complementary Medicine', because that sounds more respectable than 'alternative'. The proper term is 'alternative' because they can't be considered as 'complementary' to medicine until such time as they are shown to work. And when and if that happens, they will just be part of medicine. Until that happens they are merely snake-oil. In the words of Richard Dawkins, 'Either it is true that a medicine works or it isn't. It cannot be false in the ordinary sense but true in some "alternative" sense' (Dawkins, 2001).

How big is the problem?

The UK Universities and Colleges Admissions Service (UCAS, www.ucas.com, accessed December 2006), reveals sixty-one courses for 'complementary medicine', of which forty-five are 'Honours Bachelor of Science' degrees, eleven are two year 'foundation' degrees in science and one is an 'Honours Bachelor of Arts' (see Table 1).

Key to Table 1

Courses in CAM offered by UK universities via UCAS (December 2006). This table excludes 17 courses in 13 institutions that are not called universities but which have degree-awarding powers and are offered on UCAS. All BSc degrees are described as Honours degrees except where noted. The last column indicates the main subject areas.

Subjects: Ac, acupuncture. Ar, aromatherapy. Ay, Ayerveda. C, traditional Chinese medicine. Ch, chiropractic. He, herbal medicine.

Table 1: Alternative Medicine degrees in UK universities

	Courses	BSc	2FT	BA	Subjects
Anglia Ruskin University	2	2			Ar, R
University of Brighton	1	1			Ac
University of Central Lancashire	3	3			M, Ar, He, Ho
University of Derby	1			1	Ar, Re, M
University of East London	2	2			M, P
University of Glamorgan	1		1		N, Ch
University of Greenwich	5	4	1		Ar
Leeds Metropolitan University	1	1			Ac, He
University of Lincoln	2	2			Ac, He
Middlesex University	4	4			He, Ch, Ay
Napier University, Edinburgh[1]	3	3			Ar, R, He,
The University of Salford	3	3			R, Ho, M
Southampton Solent University	1	1			M, R
Thames Valley University	1		1		Ac, Ar, Ho
University of Westminster	14	14			N, Na, Ac, M Ho, He, C
University of Wolverhampton	1	1			Ar, R
Number of institutions	16				
Number of courses	45	41	3	1	

Key to Table 1 (cont.)

Subjects: Ho, homeopathy. N, nutrition. Na, naturopathy. R, reflexology. M, various forms of massage ('therapeutic bodywork', 'therapeutic massage', shiatsu, Indian head massage). P, pilates.

[1] Two of the three degrees are described as ordinary BSc

These courses cover many subjects, the main ones being aromatherapy, acupuncture, traditional Chinese medicine, herbal medicine, reflexology, osteopathy and homeopathy.[1] There is also therapeutic bodywork, naturopathy, nutrition, Ayurveda, Shiatsu and Qigong.[2] The most common subjects are as follows.

- Reflexology: seven courses, four of which are 'Bachelor of Science' degrees, and three three are two-year foundation degrees in 'science'.

- Homeopathy: five courses, all 'Honours Bachelor of Science' degrees in three institutions, University of Salford, Central Lancashire and Westminster.

- Traditional Chinese Medicine: six courses, all 'Honours Bachelor of Science', in three places, Middlesex University, The North East Wales Institute of Higher Education and Westminster University.

- Acupuncture: ten courses in seven places, all but one being 'Honours Bachelor of Science'.

- Aromatherapy: ten courses in eight institutions, seven being 'Honours Bachelor of Science'.

- Herbal Medicine: eight courses in six institutions, all 'Honours Bachelor of Science'.

There is one thing that is very noticeable about the institutions listed in Table 1. Every one of them is a 'post-1992' university. These are the polytechnics or colleges of higher education that were given the status of universities by John Major's government in 1992. They are mostly not very distinguished in research (though there are some notable exceptions), but they do an excellent job of teaching in many areas. It is sad that some of them have chosen to do great harm to

---

[1]   Students completing the homeopathy modules gain a 'First Aid Certificate in Homeopathy'. University of Salford,
www.chssc.salford.ac.uk/programmes/ugrad/cmhs.php

[2]   'Our vision sees therapeutic bodywork as a method for restoring and developing the natural order inherent in the human being. The word therapeutic indicates our attitude towards actively working with the client in a "healing partnership". The word bodywork relates to our use of the body as a primary resource for managing the continuum of experiences that a lifetime produces. We work with symptoms such as pain and stiffness, to postural and body use issues, to emotional and attitudinal influences. In other words working with the client and their relationship to their body to foster growth, expansion of awareness and conscious choice to bring aliveness, fluidity and enrichment to daily life.' (University of Westminster, www.wmin.ac.uk/sih/page-289). For discussion of naturopathy see www.naturowatch.org

their reputations as serious academic institutions by offering BSc degrees in subjects that are not, by any stretch of the imagination, science. Only the University of Derby is honest enough to describe its degree as a Bachelor of Arts, though in fact all the degrees are designed to lead to licences to practise CAM, so in practice it makes little difference what the degree is called.

Table 1 lists only degree courses. There is a lot more 'alternative medicine' around than that, especially if one includes university hospitals. In that case you can add to the list Glasgow, Southampton, Bristol, York, London, the Open University and quite a lot of others. In some of these cases, though, the responsibility lies with the NHS Trust, not with the university, so they fall outside the scope of this paper.

Nutrition therapy

I shall not deal with courses on nutrition in detail, because many of them are excellent. It is worth mentioning, though that some courses are no less fraudulent than most CAM. The word to look for is '*therapy*'. Its presence should ring alarm bells because it usually means that nutrition is not being used in the sense of healthy eating, but as a cure-all panacea for every illness (as long as you buy enough highly priced 'nutritional supplements' from the salesman). Two cases are worth a mention.

The University of Middlesex validates honours degrees in 'nutritional therapy' that are run entirely by a private company, the Centre for Nutrition Education and Lifestyle Management (CNELM, cnelm.co.uk). Their 2007 brochure carries the rather bizarre slogan 'Caring for and Nurturing our future Evolution through the successful support of our genetic code'.[3] Another cause for deep suspicion is that their programme includes Neuro-linguistic programming (NLP). This is an unvalidated new age method described by Stephen Barrett under the heading 'Mental Help: Procedures to Avoid'.[4] A US National Research Council committee found no significant evidence that NLP's theories are sound or that its practices are effective (Druckman, *et al.*, 1988).

The University of Bedfordshire validates external two year foundation degrees run by the 'Institute of Optimum Nutrition' (www.ion.ac.uk). Their rather optimistic motto is 'The Doctor of the future will no longer treat the human frame with drugs, but rather

[3]   www.cnelm.co.uk/Prospectus%20UG%202007.pdf
[4]   www.quackwatch.org/01QuackeryRelatedTopics/mentserv.html

will cure and prevent disease with nutrition.' Their course brochure, which starts with a large advertisement for their pill sales arm, offers 'an optional extra year's study to raise the Foundation degree to a full BSc', validated by the University of Luton.[5] The validation procedures of the University of Bedfordshire, in its previous incarnation as the University of Luton, are so poor that even the Quality Assurance Agency (see below) was able to spot them, in its 2005 report.[6] These are not 'mickey-mouse degrees'; they are much worse than that.

Sometimes degrees in vocational subjects, things like 'golf-course management', are referred to as 'mickey mouse degrees'. While it is true that, for better or worse, the nature of some universities has changed, I see nothing wrong with degrees in golf course management. They certainly have not got much intellectual content compared with the standard degrees in, say mathematics, physics or French, but they are honest. They are what it says on the label. Nobody is likely to mistake them for something they are not. The same cannot be said of degrees in homeopathy or reflexology. It is simply dishonest to award a Bachelor of Science degree in a subject that is not science. I'd better justify that statement, in case anyone doubts it.

How many of these courses are 'science'?

I'd maintain that none are. More to the point, quite a lot of CAM advocates would agree. Often it seems that CAM people suffer from a curious schizoid tendency. On one hand they are often positively antipathetic towards science, which is regarded as some sort of evil hegemony (though that certainly does not stop them spreading their views on the internet; that bit of science is apparently OK). Yet at the same time they love to use scientific-sounding words (though very often with a meaning that is different from the way the same word is used in science, or, only too often, with no discernable meaning at all). They are also eager to embrace the (rare) cases where science appears to endorse their views; at this point the antipathy to the evil hegemony vanishes in a puff of smoke. Examples are given below. This behaviour is entirely characteristic of pseudoscience, and that is precisely what most CAM is.

---

[5]   December 2007, www.ion.ac.uk/Info%20brochure%202006.pdf
[6]   www.qaa.ac.uk/reviews/reports/institutional/Luton1105/RG162UniLuton.pdf

The Prince's Foundation for Integrated Health provides a telling example. His website is well worth a look (www.fih.org.uk). It is the source of some of the wackiest advice on health that you can get anywhere. For his work on 'regulation' of CAM (see below), the Prince's Trust was given £900,000 of taxpayer's money by the Department of Health at a time when the Health Service is in financial crisis. (The question of whether it is proper for a constitutional monarch to intervene so directly in matters of public policy is one that I won't try to deal with here.) For some trenchant comments, see an editorial in the FASEB Journal, by Gerald Weissmann.

The Prince of Wales sponsored an economist, Christopher Smallwood, to produce a report on *The Role of Complementary and Alternative Medicine in the NHS* (Smallwood, 2005). Ernst has summarised some of the errors and misleading statements in this report: he comments 'I withdrew my cooperation when I became convinced that this was no honest attempt at finding the truth' (Ernst, 2006). Richard Horton, editor of the *Lancet,* said 'Let's be clear: this report contains dangerous nonsense', and 'We are losing our grip on a rational scientific medicine that has brought benefits to millions, and which is now being eroded by the complicity of doctors who should know better and a prince who seems to know nothing at all' (Horton, 2005).

Smallwood's report was widely reported in the media as advocating wider use of CAM on the NHS, but for the present purposes the really interesting thing is that it did nothing of the sort. It was very obviously sympathetic to the Prince's aims, but despite that, it actually came to the following conclusion (page 17).

> Our principle recommendation therefore is that Health Ministers should invite the National Institute of Health and Clinical Excellence (NICE) to carry out a full assessment of the cost-effectiveness of the therapies which we have identified and their potential role within the NHS in particular with a view to the closing of 'effectiveness gaps'.

What this means, in plain English, is that all their efforts to find evidence for the effectiveness of CAM produced results that were so unconvincing that they ended up by recommending that someone else (NICE) should have a go. In fact this advice has not been followed. It may not be over-sceptical to think that this is because NICE, if it were to use its normal criteria, would certainly conclude that most of the therapies were unproven or disproved. Incidentally, the Prince's Foundation also publishes 'Complementary healthcare:

a guide for patients' which shows little or no trace of the uncertainty that Smallwood found about the effectiveness of the treatments that it recommends.[7]

Next I'll cite a couple of examples of the more extreme anti-science sentiments that have been published recently.

- 'I wish to problematise the call from within biomedicine for more evidence of alternative medicine's effectiveness via the medium of the randomised clinical trial (RCT).'

- 'Ethnographic research in alternative medicine is coming to be used politically as a challenge to the hegemony of a scientific biomedical construction of evidence.'

- 'The science of biomedicine was perceived as old fashioned and rejected in favour of the quantum and chaos theories of modern physics.'

- 'In this paper, I have deconstructed the powerful notion of evidence within biomedicine … ' (Barry, 2006).

And if you thank that is bizarre, just try this one from Holmes, Murray, Peronn and Rail (Holmes *et al.*, 2006). Their paper starts thus.

Drawing on the work of the late French philosophers Deleuze and Guattari, the objective of this paper is to demonstrate that the evidence-based movement in the health sciences is outrageously exclusionary and dangerously normative with regards to scientific knowledge. As such, we assert that the evidence-based movement in health sciences constitutes a good example of microfascism at play in the contemporary scientific arena.

It is interesting to compare these quotations with this one.

Rather, they [natural scientists] cling to the dogma imposed by the long post-Enlightenment hegemony over the Western intellectual outlook, which can be summarized briefly as follows: that there exists an external world, whose properties are independent of any individual human being and indeed of humanity as a whole; that these properties are encoded in 'eternal' physical laws; and that human beings can obtain reliable, albeit imperfect and tentative, knowledge of these laws by hewing to the 'objective' procedures and epistemological strictures prescribed by the (so-called) scientific method. (Sokal, 1996)

---

[7] www.fih.org.uk/NR/rdonlyres/75C60D68-A115-42E5-A523-3DF7AC96D72/0/ComplementaryHealthcareaguideforpatients.pdf

They sound pretty similar in tone. But there is one difference. The last quotation is the opening of Alan Sokal's spoof paper which was accepted in a 'serious' journal. This episode led to publication of his book *Intellectual Impostures*, which did so much to demolish the absurd pretensions of postmodernism (well, apart from the two examples above; apparently it lives on in the murkier recesses of CAM) (Sokal and Bricmont, 1998). More relevant to our present topic is another essay by Sokal, 'Pseudoscience and Postmodernism: antagonists or fellow-travelers?', in which he argues that there is a 'curious convergence between pseudoscience and postmodernism' (Sokal, 2006).

Papers like these show an extreme form of antipathy to science (not to mention a giant chip on the shoulder), but similar attitudes can be found everywhere in the world of alternative medicine.

I'll state my position plainly. Of the topics that are the subject of the university degrees listed below in Table 2, two are self-evident nonsense, and for the rest the evidence base is far too weak for them to be the subject of degrees. I'd better justify that statement, for each of the main areas.

Homeopathy

The easiest one to deal with is homeopathy. That is simple: most of the time, the medicine contains no medicine. There is no point in beating about the bush. Homeopathy is plain fraud. The degrees on offer are shown in Table 2 below.

Table 2: Homeopathy degrees in UK universities

University of Central Lancashire	
Homoeopathic Medicine	3FT Hon BSc
The University of Salford	
Complementary Medicine and Health Sciences	3FT Hon BSc
Homeopathy in Practice (top-up)	2FT Hon BSc
University of Westminster	
Health Sciences: Homeopathy	3FT Hon BSc
Health Sciences: Homeopathy with Fdn (4 yrs)	4FT Hon BSc

Empirial evidence for homeopathy

The *Lancet* declared 'The End of Homeopathy' (yet again) in 2005 (*Lancet*, 2005) .

Surely the time has passed for selective analyses, biased reports, or further investment in research to perpetuate the homoeopathy versus allopathy debate. Now doctors need to be bold and honest with their patients about homoeopathy's lack of benefit, and with themselves about the failings of modern medicine to address patients' needs for personalised care.

And the UK's first professor of CAM, Professor Ernst, concluded there were no effects greater than placebo, and that is after almost 200 years of 'research' (Ernst, 2005). No real scientist believes it. These conclusions came 164 years after Oliver Wendell Holmes (father of the famous Supreme Court Justice, and one-time dean of Harvard Medical School) wrote his famous essay 'Homeopathy and its kindred delusions' (Holmes, 1842). Later he wrote thus.

> Some of you will probably be more or less troubled by that parody of medieval theology which finds its dogma in the doctrine of homeopathy, its miracle of transubstantiation in the mystery of its dilutions, its church in the people who have mistaken their century, and its priests in those who have mistaken their calling. (Holmes, 1871)

What is perhaps even more relevant is that it is surprisingly common for homeopaths themselves to admit that the evidence is very unconvincing (see also the reference to the Smallwood Report, above). True, they are much more likely to admit this when talking among themselves, than when engaging with scientists. For example, Verhoef, Lewith *et al.*, say

> Some of this conflict originates from the fact that many rigorous studies of CAM interventions appear to produce equivocal or negative outcomes when evaluated in the context of a conventional RCT. For instance, the Southampton research group's study on homeopathic immunotherapy for asthma was a large, well-powered and rigorous clinical trial that failed to demonstrate a difference between verum and placebo in the context of the patient's asthma. (Verhoef *et al.*, 2004)

Another example is provided by Peter Fisher, Clinical Director of the Royal London Homeopathic Hospital and homeopathic physician to the Queen. Fisher represents the more reasonable end of the homeopathic spectrum. I first came across him when I was asked by a television programme to reanalyze a trial by Fisher, Greenwood, Huskisson, Turner and Belon, which claimed a positive effect for homeopathic treatment of primary fibromyalgia (Fisher *et al.*, 1989). It turned out that a simple mistake had been made in the statistical analysis, and there were actually no effects (Colquhoun, 1990).[8] At the end of a trial that found 'no evidence that active homeopathy improves the symptoms of rheumatoid arthritis', Fisher concludes, 'It seems more important to define if homeopathists can genuinely control patients' symptoms and less relevant to have concerns about whether this is due to a "genuine" effect or to influencing the placebo response' (Fisher, 2001).

This appears to be an explicit admission that it doesn't matter whether homeopathy is better than placebo or not!

In an editorial in the journal *Homeopathy* (2006), following the *Lancet*'s declaration of 'The End of Homeopathy' in 2005, Fisher says, almost wistfully, 'And one cannot deny that the impact of allopathy on reality in recent times has been much greater than that of homeopathy' (Fisher, 2006).

And, referring to the *Lancet*'s 'wishful claim that the end of homeopathy is nigh', 'Yet Vandenbroucke's remark about changing reality is a telling one: we need to find ways to enable homeopathy to change human reality more than it has, and for the better.'

Perhaps this is wishful thinking on my own part, but these comments sound to me very like the rueful thoughts of a middle-aged Anglican vicar who, having some time ago lost his faith, nevertheless feels unable to admit it openly in case it affects his livelihood.

When challenged about the efficacy of some of his treatments, Dr Fisher referred me to the National Library for Health Complementary and Alternative Medicine Specialist Library (NeICAM, www.library.nhs.uk/cam). That library is compiled entirely by people sympathetic to CAM. As of 31 July 2006, I found twenty-seven entries relating to the assessment of homeopathy. Not a single one of these entries concludes that there is good evidence for the effectiveness of homeopathic treatment in any condition. Is this the best they can do?

Much the same conclusion can be drawn from the US equivalent (www.nccam.nih.gov/health/homeopathy), though curiously, given the enormous funding of the US National Center for Complementary and Alternative Medicine (NCCAM), this page has not been updated since April 2003. Incidentally, NCCAM has received almost a trillion dollars ($842 m). What has the US taxpayer had for

---

[8]   It is interesting that this correction has had only had seven citations (excluding self-citations) by December 2006, compared with seventy-two citations for the original paper that claimed to provide evidence for the effectiveness of homeopathy.

this money?' … it has not proved effectiveness for any "alternative" method. It has added evidence of ineffectiveness of some methods that we knew did not work before NCCAM was formed.' (Sampson, 2004).

Another example comes from the well-known homeopath, George Vithoulkas. His book *The Science of Homeopathy* [sic] is one of those recommended by the University of Westminster for its homeopathy students. On his website, one can read the following remarkable statements.

> The rejuvenation and renaissance of Homeopathy that we have been witnessing over the past thirty years seems lately doomed to take a downward turn toward a point of degeneration, confusion and, finally, even oblivion … We have had a lot of problems persuading people that Homeopathy is a Science. Now, with all this nonsense, we are once again reinforcing their arguments claiming that Homeopathy is a 'non-science'. (Vithoulkas, 2006)[9]

What is odd about this stance is that, despite their obvious doubts about the evidence, luminaries of CAM like Fisher, Lewith and Vithoulkas continue to practice it, and to defend it stoutly in public (they may even sell products in private which they themselves have deplored in public).[10] At a debate held at the Natural History Museum in London, Peter Fisher declaimed with supreme confidence 'Does homeopathy work? Yes, of course it works.'[11] No sign of public doubts there.

Most pharmacologists are too busy trying to do useful things to give a moment's thought to such nonsense. Every day pharmacologists measure curves that show response increasing as you increase the concentration of a drug. What else would you expect? Homeopaths, on the other hand maintain that the response gets bigger as you *decrease* the concentration of the drug, though they have never been able to produce a graph that shows such nonsensical behaviour. They maintain it because it says in their holy book, Hahnemann's *Organon*, not because they have seen it happening. Of course the fact that homeopathic pills, which usually contain nothing whatsoever (apart from sugar), have no effect could have been

---

[9] In the interest of accuracy, I should point out that what Vithoulkas thinks is wrong is not homeopathy itself, but modern homeopaths who have strayed from the ways of the holy book and are therefore using an ineffective form of homeopathy.

[10] See, for example, http://www.dcscience.net/improbable.html#lewith1

[11] nhm.ac.uk/nature-online/life/plants-fungi/301106homeopathy/does-homeo pathy-work.html

an advantage to patients in Hahnemann's time. It would have saved them from the physicians who often did more harm than good in 1830. But medicine has moved on, and homeopathy has not.

It would be a mistake to think that, just because homeopathic pills contain nothing but sugar that homeopathy is safe. Of course the pills themselves are totally safe, it is the homeopaths that constitute a danger to health. People like Peter Fisher are not much danger. He is clearly deeply embarrassed by fellow homeopaths who regularly do irresponsible things like recommending homeopathic pills to prevent malaria, and who recommend people not to get vaccinated (Schmidt and Ernst, 2003).[12] But the internet is overflowing with offers by homeopaths to treat really serious diseases. For example, the homeopath Robert Lee Dalpé, writes about West Nile fever.

> Homeopathy offers a unique alternative for treatment if the disease is contracted, especially in the more severe cases ... Looking over the remedies that repertorized out, I see that Lachesis came out with the strongest emphasis. Note also that Crotalus horridus is there as well. This indicates to me that snake remedies in general may be useful for this disease. So I have added Vipera as the 22nd remedy even though it did not repertorize down, but exists in one of the two larger rubrics. So we must consider all snake remedies here. A technique of prescribing Sheilagh Creasy once taught me was to 'switch snakes' as required in a case. So, all snakes are 'on the table', as it were.[13]

This sort of dangerous gobbledygook is what you get when you abandon reason. Incidentally, Sheilagh Creasy, mentioned here, is a member of the team that teaches the homeopathy 'BSc' at the University of Westminster.[14]

The analogy between homeopathy and religious sect is remarkable.[15] That includes the charismatic leader, the holy book and also the internecine strife so characteristic of religious sects. Here is an example from Dr Richard H. Pitcairn, May 2002, Past President of the Academy of Veterinary Homeopathy in the USA.[16]

---

[12] The facts about malaria prevention were revealed by Sense About Science (http://www.senseaboutscience.org.uk/index.php/site/project/71/) and the BBC Newsnight programme
(http://news.bbc.co.uk/1/hi/programmes/newsnight/5178122.stm).
[13] http://www.onlinehomeopath.com/westnile.shtml, December 2006.
[14] www.wmin.ac.uk/sih/page-59
[15] National Council Against Health Fraud, December 2006,
www.ncahf.org/pp/homeop.html
[16] Grundlagen & Praxis, International Discussion: basis of homeopathy, December 2006; www.grundlagen-praxis.de/debatte/englisch/short.pdf

> ... I too have been very concerned about the direction homeopathy is taking. It seems that so many people want to practice in contradiction to the principles Hahnemann so carefully discovered. It is presenting as 'progress' but my experience is that these approaches are ineffective as so many of my colleagues that have gone to practitioners of the 'new methods' are not helped at all.

Homeopaths are a bit like creationists: they prefer to rely on ancient dogma rather than to think. It is the lazy approach.

What are students taught on homeopathy degree degrees?

So what are students actually taught? Most academics are happy to tell you what they teach, and many course materials are freely available to anyone. But not homeopaths. The University of Central Lancashire turned down (three times) a request under the Freedom of Information Act 2000 to make available some of the teaching materials used on their 'BSc' in homeopathy. Clearly they are embarrassed by the idea that the public (who paid for them) might see what they teach. (I am still waiting for result of an appeal to the Information commissioner.)

You can get a good idea from what goes on from the examination question shown in Figure 1 (below). This exam was set by the University of Westminster in 2005 (I'm not giving anything away; past papers are available to students on the University website).

What does all this mean? Consider the words 'Miasmatic nature'. The miasmatic theory held that diseases like cholera and plague were spread by foul air, known as miasmas. This theory originated in the Middle Ages and lasted until the middle of the nineteenth century. It was used, for example, to explain the spread of cholera in London. The word 'miasm' was used in a similar sense by homeopaths, 'miasms' being the source of chronic diseases. Here are the words of the master.

> The true natural chronic diseases are those that arise from a chronic miasm, which when left to themselves, and unchecked by the employment of those remedies that are specific for them, always go on increasing and growing worse, notwithstanding the best mental and corporeal regimen, and torment the patient to the end of his life with ever aggravated sufferings. These are the most numerous and greatest scourges of the human race; for the most robust constitution, the best regulated mode of living and the most vigorous energy of the vital force are insufficient for their eradication. (Hahnemann, 1833)

Figure 1

Cavendish Campus

School of Integrated Health

BSc Complementary Therapies Scheme

Module 3CTH 502

Homœopathic Materia Medica 2A

Module Leader: Mark Paine

Section B
Answer **ONE** question
Total marks available 50.

KALI CARBONICUM and **TUBERCULINUM** are both in the rubric "obstinate, headstrong." (*Synthesis*)

Explain why these two remedies appear in this rubric. Clearly differentiate between them in relation to the rubric, focusing on their physical, general and mental/emotional picture.

OR

PSORINUM and **SULPHUR** are *Psoric remedies.*

a) Discuss the ways in which the symptoms of these remedies reflect their miasmatic nature. *(35 marks)*

b) Define and differentiate between the features of the two remedies. *(15 marks)*

According to Hahnemann there are three miasms: 'psora', 'sycosis' and 'syphilis'.[17] Later homeopaths added for example the Tubercular, Cancer and Aids.[18]

---

[17] Psora, psoric, miasm [Lat. *psora, psorae* — Pliny: itch, mange]. Samuel Hahnemann, the founder of homeopathy considered Psora as the most important miasm and the psoric miasm as the fundamental cause of disease.
See also
http://www.lyghtforce.com/homeopathyonline/issue2/educate3.html
http://en.wikipedia.org/wiki/Classical_homeopathy#Miasms
[18] www.homeopathy.healthspace.eu/regular/homeopathy.php#Miasms

Of course, the problem of cholera was solved when it was shown by John Snow, in 1854, that cholera was spread through contaminated water, not 'miasmas', and the mechanism became clear when Robert Koch discovered the micro-organism that causes cholera in 1883. Science moved on, and, with a lot of hard work, discovered something true about the causes of disease. The superstitious ideas about miasmas vanished. Well, they vanished for all rational people, but homeopathy remained stuck firmly in the 1830s. Figure 1 shows that the homeopaths of the University of Westminster still think it appropriate to set exams on miasms in 2006. You couldn't make it up if you tried.

I'll finish with a couple of quotations from one of the wittiest denunciations of homeopathy I've encountered.[19]

> When Hahnemann speaks of 'Psora, the Mother of all true chronic diseases,' he creates a new version of Lilith, a demoness of disease, conquerable with the Vitalism that is likewise an invisible spirit. He further taught of the authority of 'Health, a spiritual power, autocracy [or] vital force.' This Spiritual Power also known as Vitalism is the 'good' spirit of the universe at odds with Psora the 'bad' spirit in the universe.

> I have tried to find a nuttier popular health fad than homeopathy and there is none.

> Hahnemann, the L. Ron Hubbard of his day, even claimed that reading his book was sufficient to frighten away many of the Psora 'itches' or demonic spirits) inhabiting sick people's bodies, and he aggressively sold the book to patients as a 'medicine' in and of itself.

This stuff is, it seems, called 'science' by the University of Westminster (see Figure 1).

On the nonsense of dilutions and the 'memory of water'

I'll repeat, briefly, the well-known fact that many homeopathic medicines contain no trace, not a single molecule, of the ingredient on the label. The commonly used 30C dilution means dilution by a factor of $100^{30} = 10^{60}$. That means that, on average, there is one molecule in a sphere with a diameter of 1.46×10^8 km7 which is close to the distance from the earth to the sun. That's hard to swallow. Put another way, 1g of starting material will produce 10^{60} g of the final dilution. That is of the order of the mass of the observable universe.[20] No wonder the profits of the homeopathic industry are so big. Even a single

[19] www.paghat.com/fothergill.html
[20] e.g. http://curious.astro.cornell.edu/question.php?number=342

feather would be enough to make a vast number of pills (that is not a joke, by the way; you can buy homeopathic owl feathers).

Many homeopaths like to say (misleadingly) in public that they use 'very high dilutions', but most will admit in private that any dilution greater than about 12C is unlikely to contain a single molecule of the material on the label. That is the point when the really zany pseudoscience starts. The structure of water has been studied intensively by serious scientists. It is true that water molecules will form structures round a solute but at room temperature, thermal motion of water molecules ensures that these structures are very short-lived, of the order of picoseconds. One of the most recent estimates is even faster, in the femtosecond range. Cowan *et al.* conclude, 'Our results highlight the efficiency of energy redistribution within the hydrogen-bonded network, and that liquid water essentially loses the memory of persistent correlations in its structure within 50 fs' (Cowan *et al.*, 2005).

That is a pretty lousy shelf life.

How do homeopaths escape this? Here are two laughable attempts.

Peter Fisher, at the end of the debate at the Natural History Museum said, 'It's true, If you take a homeopathic medicine to an analytical chemist and say 'What's in here?', he'll say it's lactose, water and alcohol. Which is quite true.'[21]

So far, so good. But he then went on to say that his gigabyte memory stick would, according to a chemist, be made almost entirely of silica with trace impurities of boron and phosphorus. 'Yet it can hold a lot of information'. 'So this property of simple chemicals storing large amounts of information is actually commonplace. What actually is so implausible about this? The possibility that water actually stores information and then transmits it to the body.'

The analogy is so obviously naive that it needs no comment. But at least it isn't pretentious. That can't be said of many attempts.

George Vithoulkas, author of *The Science of Homeopathy*, makes this attempt. 'Just as physics moved from the Newtonian era into the concepts of modern physics, the field of medicine is slowly beginning to understand the realms of energy fields in the human body.'

That of course is simply not true. There isn't the slightest reason to believe in the existence of the 'energy fields' so beloved by quacks. One can read endless tedious invocations of relativity, quantum entanglement by homeopaths most of whom could probably not be

[21] See above note 11.

able to differentiate e^x, never mind understand quantum theory. It is all pure pseudoscientific gobbledygook. It is also the subject of Bachelor of Science degrees at three UK universities, as well as endless courses and diplomas.

The result of having a homeopathy degree in a multi-faculty university is that you have one department teaching that effect increases with dose (backed by endless observations) and another department teaching exactly the opposite (backed by nothing but a holy book). In fact some students are taught both conflicting views, so 'on Mondays and Thursdays (for example) the students must believe that response increases with dose, but on Tuesdays and Fridays they are called upon to believe that response decreases with dose.'[22]

Perhaps the real clincher came after *Nature* published a collection of attacks on the incursion of homeopathy into universities.[23] After this appeared, I debated the question on a BBC television news programme with with Dr Peter Fisher. The interview concluded thus.

> *Riz Lateef* (presenter): Dr Fisher, could you ever see it [homeopathy] as a science degree in the future?

> *Dr Peter Fisher:* I would hope so. I wouldn't deny that a lot of scientific research needs to be done, and I would hope that in the future it would have a scientific basis. I have to say that at the moment that basis isn't comprehensive. To that extent I would agree with Professor Colquhoun.

So we are now in the absurd position that the UK's most senior homeopath agrees that there is not a sufficient scientific basis to make homeopathy a BSc degree, but vice-chancellors of universities do not agree.

Reflexology

Reflexology is just foot massage, and there is nothing wrong with that if it makes you happy. Unfortunately the massage is accompanied by a lot of gobbledygook. It is alleged, without a fragment of evidence, that particular areas on the foot are linked to other areas of the body. You can see the hilarious charts in many places.[24] The Association of Reflexologists, after giving a long list of conditions for

[22] http://dcscience.net/?p=83
[23] *Nature*, 446 (2007), 373– 4. See also http://dcscience.net/?p=19
[24] e.g. The Modern Institute of Reflexology, December 2006,
http://www.reflexologyinstitute.com/reflex_chart.php

which it claims (falsely) that 'Reflexology has been shown to be effective for', then says (more realistically) that 'Reflexology does not claim to cure, diagnose or prescribe' (www.reflexology.org). So what *does* it do? Consider this bit of sheer fantasy.

> Reflexologists believe that sensitive and trained hands can detect tiny deposits and imbalances in the feet. And by working on these points the reflexologist can release blockages and restore the free flow of energy to the whole body. it is believed that nerve endings are unable to transmit their impulses because of crystalline deposits that build up and block their pathway. Reflexology is believed to clear these crystalline deposits.

Reflexology lies firmly in the realm of pseudoscience. To give Bachelor of Science degrees to people who manage to memorise such fantasies is the height of irresponsibility.

Acupuncture

Unlike the cases of homeopathy and reflexology, there is nothing inherently absurd about acupuncture. It is pretty obvious that sticking needles into your body will produce signals in the brain. Of course that does not mean that sticking needles into you will benefit any particular medical condition. There is a bit of suggestive evidence that it may help a few conditions but the evidence is very thin indeed for a practice that is so widely used. What is really objectionable about acupuncture is the mumbo jumbo that accompanies the needles. Take a typical exposition of the 'principles' of acupuncture.[25]

'There are 14 major avenues of energy flowing through the body. These are known as meridians.'

- The energy that moves through the meridians is called Qi.
- Think of Qi as 'The Force'. It is the energy that makes a clear distinction between life and death.
- Acupuncture needles are gently placed through the skin along various key points along the meridians. This helps rebalance the Qi so the body systems work harmoniously.

I suppose, to the uneducated, this language sounds a bit like that of physics. But it is not. The words have no discernable meaning whatsoever. In any case, there is some empirical evidence that it

[25]　December 2006, http://www.anewdayhealingarts.com/acupuncture.htm; see also Wikipedia http://en.wikipedia.org/wiki/Acupuncture .

doesn't matter where you put the needles; whatever effects you get are much the same wherever you are pierced. So much for 'ancient wisdom'. One shouldn't really be surprised: the main characteristic of ancient wisdom is that most of it is dead wrong.

No respectable university could subject students to this sort of mumbo-jumbo, pretending that it is science.

Herbal medicine

Herbal medicine is in a different category from homeopathy, reflexology and acupuncture. It is pharmacology, not black magic. Several useful medicines came originally from plants and there could well be more waiting to be found. The only thing that distinguishes 'herbal medicine' from pharmacology is that the former consists, almost entirely of things that are not yet proved to work, and are not standardised. To offer a 'BSc' degree in unproven treatments (see Table 1) is absurd.

First remember that plants did not evolve for the benefit of humans. Natural selection ensures that plants, like every other living thing, evolve in a way that maximises their own chance of survival. To ensure this, plants should be as toxic as possible to anything that might eat them. The more harm a plant does to humans, the better its chance of survival. It is sheer luck that a few of the toxic principles evolved by plants occasionally turn out to be useful.

A pharmacological example may make matters clearer. The 24th edition of Martindale's *Extra Pharmacopoeia* (1958) describes *Digitalis Leaf* (B.P., I.P.), also known as Digit. Fol.; Digitalis; Foxglove Leaf; Feuille de Digitale; Fingerhutblatt; Hoja de digital. It was defined as 'the dried leaves of Digitalis purpurea (Scrophulariaceae).'

At that time it was sometimes prescribed as *Prepared Digitalis (BP)*, which is 'Digitalis leaf reduced to powder, no part being rejected, and biologically assayed the strength being stated in units per g. For therapeutic purposes it must be adjusted to contain 10 units in 1 g.'

Sometimes foxglove leaf was prescribed as *Tincture of Digitalis (B.P., I.P.)*.

> It may be made from unstandardised leaf, the tincture being subsequently biologically assayed, or it may be made from prepared digitalis, using a quantity containing 1000 units per litre, by percolation or maceration, with alcohol (70 %). It contains 1 unit per ml. I.P. allows also 1 unit per g. Dose: 0.3 to 1 ml. (5 to 15 minims).

Although these preparations are now totally defunct, they were still better than the sort of thing that is now advocated by herbalists. Why? They were better because they were standardised.

Foxglove leaves contain several chemical compounds that are useful in certain forms of heart failure. But the margin of safety is quite low. Take a bit too much and it kills you not cures you. One batch of foxglove leaves will contain different amounts of active compounds from the last batch, and that endangered patients.

From the 1930s onwards, pharmacologists and statisticians went to great efforts to develop methods of biological assay that overcame this problem. An international standard digitalis leaf sample was established. Every new batch had to be assayed against this standard, and diluted to a fixed level of biological activity. This ensured that each batch of digitalis powder had the same biological potency as the last batch. It was a great pharmacological advance in its time, though of course it did involve the use of animals for the biological assay.

All this was solved when the active principles were purified from the foxglove leaves. There was no longer any need to use animals for biological assays. The right amount of pure digoxin or digitoxin could be weighed out.

Herbalists want to go back to the times before 1930, using impure *and* unstandardised plant extracts. In this case, and all others I can think of, there is not the slightest reason to think that the impure mixture in the leaf is any better than the purified active principles. Of course there *could* be such cases. But that is just idle speculation

You cannot base a Bachelor of Science degree on idle speculations.

Traditional Chinese medicine

Traditional Chinese medicine is much like herbal medicine. It differs in two obvious ways. It does not restrict itself to plants but includes things like shark fin, tiger bones, rhinoceros horn (though not, as far as I know, eye of newt or toe of frog). It also differs in having in being overlaid with layers of magic; the same sort of tedious talk about 'Qi', 'Yin and Yang' that acupuncturists like to mouth, but which has no discernable meaning.

Since the medicines do contain something (unlike homeopathy) it is not inconceivable that they might work, but the few well conducted clinical trials that have been done have failed, with very few exceptions, to show anything much that is useful.

Chinese medicine has also suffered from political promotion in China, for reasons of nationalism (and perhaps to save money). There it is still an accepted part of the health system, rather than, as in the West, being restricted to the lunatic fringe. Even in China, though, there is no government-promoted 'Chinese Physics'. Perhaps that is simply because it is a lot easier to tell whether an electronic toy works than it is to tell if a medicine works.

Like herbal medicine, Chinese 'remedies' are totally unstandardised and there have been many reports of toxicity either through overdose, or as a result of contamination with toxic compounds.

It is hard to see why, in 2006, this sort of mediaeval approach to medicine continues to exist. It is harder still to understand why any university should consider it an appropriate subject for a Bachelor of Science degree.

Next I shall consider why it has not yet vanished.

The accreditation of degrees and the Quality Assurance Agency

The tradition of Staff Xmas Dinners at Poppleton is one of the few elements of university life that has not been validated by competent authorities. To remedy this situation, the specially constituted Xmas Dinner Committee has issued the following guidelines.

All members of staff who wish to attend such functions are urged to participate in one of the special Staff Development Workshops on Social Interaction that are being held every weekday evening in the Staff Development Complex.

All departments intending to hold a Staff Xmas Dinner are required to submit a statement of Dining Aims and Outcomes and indicate the manner in which learning outcomes will be assessed. All diners will be required to complete a Post Dining Questionnaire that includes learning outcomes and a TQA (turkey quality assessment). (Taylor, 2006.)

Laurie Taylor's parody captures beautifully the tide of bureaucracy that has engulfed universities. It would not be so bad if the bureaucracy accomplished anything useful, but most of it doesn't. There are two mechanisms that are intended to ensure that university degrees reach a satisfactory standard. First, courses must be accredited before they can run. Once they are running they are subject to scrutiny by the Quality Assurance Agency for Higher Education (QAA).

Nothing illustrates more perfectly the total failure of both mechanisms than the existence of 'BSc' degrees in subjects that are not science. In fact it is worse than that. The accreditation mechanism and the QAA actually appear to endorse courses that might otherwise have been treated with the derision they deserve.

Accreditation

'Accreditation' is an elaborate bureaucratic process that is designed to perpetuate the fallacy that degrees are of high quality and comparable in different institutions. What happens in real life, of course, is that courses in things like homeopathy or naturopathy are accredited by homeopaths and naturopaths. Barmy courses get barmy assessors so the process of accreditation provides no protection whatsoever against courses in homeopathy (or astrology, or voodoo).

The Quality Assurance Agency for Higher Education (QAA)

The QAA declares that 'We safeguard and help to improve the academic standards and quality of higher education in the UK.' For this job we, the taxpayers, pay them £11.5 million annually. One might expect that they would have noticed that some universities are awarding 'BSc' degrees in subjects that are not, by any stretch of the imagination, science. But in that expectation you would be disappointed.

The QAA report on the University of Westminster courses awards a perfect score for 'Curriculum Design, Content and Organisation'. It did not worry the assessors that the content consists of early nineteenth century myths, not science. As with all academic reports, the view one takes of the opinions depends on who expressed those opinions, but the authors of the report are anonymous.

The chief executive of the QAA, Peter Williams, pointed out to me that it would be unacceptable for the QAA to interfere with university autonomy, and it would indeed be a bad thing if we were told what to do by a government agency. But if, as seems to be the case, non-interference extends to giving high scores to the content of nonsense degrees, it is hard to see what use the agency can be. It should be abandoned if it can't do better than that. In fairness, it has been given a job that is impossible to do. The real blame lies with vice-chancellors.

Regulatory agencies

In addition to the mechanisms that are meant to regulate the standards of degrees, but fail to do so, there also some mechanisms that are meant to regulate CAM itself. There is some regulatory legislation and there is the Medicines and Healthcare products Regulatory Agency (MHRA). Both have done more harm than good because both have chosen to ignore the one vital question, 'does the medicine work?' The only result of this sort of regulation is to give the impression of government approval to treatments that mostly don't work. There can be no more graphic illustration of the age of spin and delusion. How does such a ludicrous state of affairs come about? As far as one can tell, it is a result of both political and royal pressure, and of commercial pressure from the CAM industry. The health of the homeopathic industry is clearly more important to the government than the health of people. The recent decision of the MHRA to allow untrue labels to be put on homeopathic pills and herbal medicines has not done much to help the cause of reason. This decision resulted in annulment debate in the House of Lords, and was condemned by the Royal Society, the Medical Research Council, the Academy of Medical Sciences, the Royal College of Pathologists, the Biosciences Federation (which represents forty affiliated societies), the Physiological Society and the British Pharmacological Society.

The reason that all these attempts at regulation have failed so badly is that none of them, incredibly, has thought it necessary to consider whether the medicines that they are meant to regulate actually work. Once again, you couldn't make it up if you tried.

The dilemmas of alternative medicine

Hard experience has shown that anyone who deplores witchcraft in medicine is immediately accused of neglecting the human side of medicine.

First, then, I must say there is nothing wrong with holism; every conventional physician is taught to treat the patient as a whole, and does so insofar as time and skill allow. And there is absolutely nothing wrong with the placebo effect. If a patient says they feel better, then they do feel better, and it doesn't matter to the patient whether that was the result of a kind word, or a green coloured sugar pill. Medical science has achieved marvels in the last 150 years. Just think of life without anaesthetics (general and local), antibiotics or artificial hips. That being said, it must be admitted that there is a great deal that medicine cannot do. It can do nothing for the common cold, and precious little for back pain. Most pharmacology (antibiotics excepted) is palliative rather than curative. If, as is only too often the case, there is nothing much that a physician can do for a patient, then anything that can be done to support the patient, to make them happier, is a good thing. BUT it should be done as honestly as possible. This leads to several very real dilemmas.[26]

The definition dilemma

- Once any treatment is shown beyond doubt to be effective, it ceases to be 'alternative' and becomes just like any other part of medical knowledge. That means that 'alternative medicine' must consist entirely of unproven treatments.

The lying dilemma

- Suppose that a treatment owes *all* its effectiveness to the placebo effect, e,g. homeopathy. In some people, at least, the placebo effect is quite real. It may be a genuine physical response, though one that does not depend on any activity of the drug, or other treatment, though quite often it is probably merely the passage of time that gives the illusion of effectiveness.

- If placebo effects are real, it would be wrong to deprive patients of them, if there is nothing more effective available. For example, if terminal cancer patients say they feel better after having their feet massaged by a 'reflexologist', why should they not have that small pleasure?

- If the foregoing argument is granted, then it follows that it would be our duty to maximise the placebo effect. In the absence of specific research, it seems reasonable to suppose that people who are susceptible to placebo effects will get the best results if their treatment is surrounded by as much impressive mumbo jumbo as possible.

- This suggests that, in order to maximise the placebo effect, it will be important to lie to the patient as much as possible, and certainly to disguise from them the fact that, for example, their homeopathic pill contains nothing but lactose.

- Therein lies the dilemma. The whole trend in medicine has been to be more open with the patient and to tell them the truth. Physicians are no longer allowed to prescribe a placebo if they call it, honestly, a placebo, but they are allowed to prescribe them if they lie to the patient (and quite possibly to themselves

---

[26] e.g. http://dcscience.net/?page_id=10

too) and call it a homeopathic pill. To maximise the benefit of alternative medicine, it is necessary to lie to the patient as much as possible.

As if telling lies to patients were not enough, the dilemma has another aspect, which is also almost always overlooked. Who trains CAM practitioners? Are the trainers expected to tell their students the same lies? Certainly that is the normal practice at the moment. Consider some examples.

The training dilemma

If a foot massage makes patients feel better, then they should have it. But then it might be thought necessary to hire professional foot massagers who have been trained in 'reflexology'. If the medicine-free sugar pills of the homeopath produce a good placebo effect then it might be thought necessary to hire a professional homeopath, skilled in the mumbo-jumbo of that subject. But who does the training? It cannot be expected that any respectable university will provide a course that preaches the mumbo jumbo of meridians, energy flows and Qi as though they were science

How are we to escape from these dilemmas? The lying dilemma could be solved if effort were put into looking for ways of giving the best possible supportive care for patients for whom nothing else can be done, without resorting to ancient gobbledygook and with lies kept, at least, to a minimum.

It is the training dilemma that is the main concern of this article. It would be solved automatically if people were to abandon treatments based on superstition and myth, but there is little chance of that happening soon, given the power and the mendacity with which superstition and myth are marketed. But there are hopeful signs that the NHS may be persuaded to abandon useless treatment. It would help enormously if regulatory agencies and the Advertising Standards Authority insisted on honest advertising and labelling. At the moment they do not, but it is not impossible that they might be persuaded to do so.

In the end, though, it is vice-chancellors of universities who must take responsibility for what is taught. If they come to realise the harm that they do to the prestige of their universities by awarding Bachelor of Science degrees in subjects that are not science, one problem at least will be solved.

References

Barry, C.A. (2006), 'The role of evidence in alternative medicine: contrasting biomedical and anthropological approaches', in *Social Science and Medicine*, 62, 2464-57.

Colquhoun, D. (1990), 'Reanalysis of a clinical trial of a homoeopathic treatment of Fibrositis', in *Lancet*, 336, 441–2.

Cowan, M.L., Bruner, B.D., Huse, N., Dwyer, J.R., Chugh, B., Nibbering, E.T., *et al.* (2005), 'Ultrafast memory loss and energy redistribution in the hydrogen bond network of liquid H_2O', in *Nature*, 10, 434: 199–202.

Dawkins, R. (2001), from the foreword to *Snake Oil* by John Diamond (Vantage).

Druckman, D. and Swets, J.A. (1988), *Enhancing Human Performance* (National Academy Press).

Ernst, E. (2005), 'Is homeopathy a clinically valuable approach?', in *Trends Pharmacological Science*, 26, 547–8.

Ernst, E. (2006), 'The Smallwood report: method or madness?', in *British Journal of General Practice*, 56, 64–5.

Fisher, P., Greenwood, A., Huskisson, E.C., Turner, P., Belon, P. (1989), 'Effect of homoeopathic treatment on Fibrositis (primary fibromyalgia)', in *British Medical Journal*, 299, 365–6.

Fisher, P. (2006), 'Changing reality', in *Homeopathy*, 95:1, 1–2.

Fisher, P. and Scott, D.L. (2001), 'A randomized controlled trial of homeopathy in Rheumatoid Arthritis', in *Rheumatology (Oxford)*, 40:9, 1052–5.

Hahnemann, S. (1833), *Organon of Medicine* (5th edn), available at
http://www.homeopathyhome.com/reference/organon/organon.html

Holmes, O.W. (1842), *Homeopathy and its kindred delusions*.
Full text at
http://www.quackwatch.org/01QuackeryRelatedTopics/holmes.html

Holmes, O.W. (1871), *Medical Essays. The Young Practitioner*, A Valedictory Address delivered to the Graduating Class of the Bellevue Hospital College, March 2, 1871.

Holmes, D., Murray, S.J., Perron, A., Rail, G. (2006), 'Deconstructing the evidence-based discourse in health sciences: truth, power and fascism', in *International Journal of Evidence-Based Healthcare*, 4, 180–6.

Horton, R. (2005), 'Rational medicine is being undermined', in the *Guardian* 8 Aug 2005,
http://www.guardian.co.uk/letters/story/0,,1587525,00.html

Lancet (2005). Editorial, 'The End of Homeopathy', in the *Lancet*, 336, 690.

Martindale, *Extra Pharmacopoeia* (pub. details)

Prince's Foundation for Integrated Health, December 2007.

Sampson, W.I. (2002), 'Why the National Center for Complementary and Alternative Medicine (NCCAM) should be defunded',
http://www.quackwatch.org/01QuackeryRelatedTopics/nccam.html

Schmidt, K. and Ernst, E. (2003), 'MMR vaccination advice over the internet', in *Vaccine*, 21:11–12,1044–7.

Sokal, A.D. (1996), 'Transgressing the boundaries: towards a transformative hermeneutics of quantum gravity', in *Social Text*, 46/47 (*Science Wars*), 217–52.

Sokal, A.D. (2006), 'Pseudoscience and postmodernism: antagonists or fellow-travelers?', in *Archaeological Fantasies* , ed. G.G. Fagan (Routledge, an imprint of Taylor & Francis Books Ltd).

Sokal, A.D. and Bricmont, J. (1998), *Intellectual Impostures* (Profile Books; new edn Economist Books, 2003).

Smallwood, C. (2005), 'The role of complementary and alternative medicine in the NHS'. The Prince's Foundation for Integrated Health, http://www.fih.org.uk/NR/rdonlyres/214DE09D-0BD6-4CAB-908C-33E2B71093AE/0/Smallwood.pdf

Taylor, L. (2006), in *Times Higher Educational Supplement*, 14 November 2006.

Verhoef, M.J., Lewith, G., Ritenbaugh, C., Thomas, K., Boon, H., Fønnebø, V. (2004), 'Whole systems research: moving forward', in *Focus on Alternative and Complementary Therapies (FACT)*, 9, 87–90.

Vithoulkas, G. (2006), 'Is Hahnemannian Homeopathy doomed to go in to oblivion again?', International Academy of Classical Homeopathy. http://www.vithoulkas.com/EN/homeopathy-doomed_oblivion.html

Vithoulkas (no date), *The Science of Homeopathy*.

Weissmann, G. (2006), 'Homeopathy: Holmes, Hogwarts, and the Prince of Wales', in *The FASEB Journal*, 20 (2006), 1755–8. http://www.fasebj.org/cgi/content/full/20/11/1755).

Bruce G. Charlton

Healing but not Curing

Alternative medical therapies as valid New Age spiritual healing practices

I argue here that alternative therapies should be seen as valid New Age spiritual healing practices, but as such they cannot be integrated with orthodox medicine or science.

I wish to suggest a new way of considering alternative and complementary therapies. Common attitudes towards alternative therapies tend to be polarized into two extreme views. The first view is that alternative therapies do-good for many people and so they should therefore be integrated with orthodox medicine. The second, and opposite view, is that alternative therapies are worthless or harmful and they should be ignored or eradicated. A third position is that alternative therapies may or may not do-good, and this should be decided using the methods of medical science.

I believe that all three of these views are mistaken. My interpretations is; 1. Alternative therapies indeed do good for many people. 2 From a strictly medical perspective they are worthless. 3. Alternative therapies should not be integrated with orthodox medicine. 4. They cannot meaningfully be investigated using the methods of medical science. Because alternative therapies do not 'cure' disease, they have no role in orthodox medicine; and because they are explained non-scientifically, they cannot be evaluated using the criteria of medical science.

My suggestion is that alternative therapies should be regarded as spiritual practices, linked to the phenomenon of New Age spirituality. This is a valid benefit in the modern world. But the benefit is psychological not medical. Alternative therapies are about making people feel better ('healing') not about mending their dysfunctional brains and bodies ('curing').

Differences between alternative therapy and orthodox medicine

I would define alternative therapies in terms of them having non-scientific explanations. In so far as a therapy does have a biological explanation, I would regard that therapy as simply part of orthodox medicine. The crucial difference between orthodox and alternative therapies is therefore that alternative medical systems have non-scientific explanations based on spiritual, mystical, legendary or otherwise intuitively-appealing insights.

This difference between orthodox and alternative medicine can be illustrated with an example. In orthodox medicine, the illness of 'hypertension' or high blood pressure is explained in terms of a mass of inter-linked biological knowledge concerning the structure and function of the human body including heart and arteries and the functional relationship between blood pressure and diseases such as stroke. Treatment of hypertension is based on a detailed scientific understanding of how the heart and arteries are regulated by the nervous system, and how this can be modified using drugs. The fact that orthodox therapies are embedded in standard biological science is what makes them scientifically testable.

By contrast, acupuncture is based around the existence of meridians, which are structures described in historic medical and religious literature but not detectable using scientific equipment. If the theory of acupuncture does not actually contradict modern biological science, then it has nothing to do with it.

In homoeopathy, the mechanism of action is based on a 'magical' form of reasoning — the 'law of similars', or like-cures-like — which has no basis in modern therapeutics. Another homeopathic principle, that of increasing potency of a medicine with increasing dilution (so long as dilution is done in a particular way called succussion) is in contradiction with modern chemistry. So the theories of homoeopathy flatly contradict modern pharmacology.

And in chiropractic medicine, the presumed spinal vertebral subluxations which are supposed to cause disease are not visible using imaging technologies such as X-rays or MRI scans. The key diagnostic features of chiropractic medicine are therefore based on a theory derived from intuition, rather than science.

Yet acupuncture, homeopathy and chiropractic are among the most professionalized of alternative therapies — the explanatory theories for crystal healing or aromatherapy are even more imaginative and less scientific. The conclusion is that alternative medical systems are disconnected from the knowledge and practices of modern science.

Alternative therapies are similarly disconnected from orthodox medicine. Despite many decades or centuries of experience, there is not one clear-cut instance in which any alternative therapy is unequivocally effective and indicated for any particular disease or symptom. There are no cures of the otherwise incurable—nobody dragged back from certain death in the way that has happened many millions of times with antibiotics and steroids. Severed limbs are not re-attached to bodies, nor diseased internal organs extracted, nor (despite the misleading political propaganda for acupuncture) can reliable anaesthesia be induced.

It is noticeable that the only positive trials in alternative therapies have been reported for conditions characterized by very unpredictable and reversible symptoms such as occur in hay fever, rhinitis, asthma, eczema, back pain, arthritic pain, migraine, chronic fatigue, post-operative ileus, and multiple sclerosis. These are conditions where it is hard to prove that anything works, where factors such as the placebo effect play a large role and where subtle biases or errors in experimental design (and publication) can most easily generate falsely positive results.

In order to design experiments to test a therapy, the therapy needs a scientific explanation; and when this is lacking there are problems—even in orthodox medicine. When orthodox medical treatments have proven effectiveness in the usual randomized clinical trials but lack an accepted scientific explanation, then the results of these trials tend to be regarded with suspicion. For example, electro-convulsive or 'shock' therapy (ECT) in psychiatry has undergone many clinical trials demonstrating its effectiveness and safety, yet it remains unpopular largely due to the fact that there has never been a widely accepted scientific explanation for why this therapy is effective. Because medical scientists cannot agree on how ECT works, it is hard to know whether it really is working, or even whether it might be doing more harm than good.

Medical treatments need scientifically plausible explanations for their actions. When a truly effective intervention emerges within an alternative medical system, its benefits therefore need to be re-explained using 'orthodox' theories in order that it can be evaluated and before doctors can be confident about prescribing it.

St John's Wort (*hypericum*) is a safe and effective antidepressant herbal medication as confirmed by a wide range of research methods including clinical trials, animal experiments and laboratory techniques. In my opinion, St John's Wort is an excellent orthodox antidepressant; and the only plausible reason why it is not by now out-selling the selective serotonin reuptake-inhibitors (such as fluoxetine/ 'Prozac'), is that the herb cannot be patented, and so it does not justify the huge expense of an international marketing effort.

The herb has been slotted into orthodox medicine by treating it as essentially interchangeable with conventional antidepressants and anti-anxiety drugs, and using the same research theories and methods developed for these orthodox medical therapies. This links St John's Wort into standard scientific modes of explanation for drugs and, in principle, enables the herb to be examined using a wide range of scientific methods.

What is New Age spirituality, and why do alternative therapies fit into its definition?

I have said that alternative therapies are not a part of science, but should instead be considered part of New Age spirituality — however, the meaning of 'New Age' may require further explanation.

New Age spirituality is a very broadly-defined term which tends to be used to refer to people who overtly adopt an 'alternative' or 'green' lifestyle, which evolved from the hippies of the late 1960s. And surveys have shown that alternative therapies are indeed very popular among this group. But the typical New Age style of spirituality is, in fact, much more widespread than this minority counter-culture fringe, indeed New Age practices involve perhaps the majority of the population in modernizing societies.

The New Age focuses on subjective psychological states such as integration, authenticity and self-expression. If traditional religion can be seen as a combination of spirituality and church (i.e. a formal institutional structure) then New Age can be conceptualized as individual spirituality separate from churches. In the past, spirituality was controlled by churches, and the forms and practices of spirituality were restricted. New Age really is something new, a product of modern individuals, and the lifestyle was not possible in earlier and less complex stages of society.

Essentially, New Age consists of individuals pursuing their own spiritual goals in their own way. They make evaluations based upon what kinds of spiritual benefit they want, and what is effective in achieving these benefits. A New Age 'seeker' needs to be free to choose (liberal democracy), have a sufficiently large range of choices (market economy), requires access to these choices (mass media) and can then express the resulting behaviours in terms of an individual and unique 'lifestyle' such as their conversation or writings, style of dress, purchases, hobbies and social activities (this requires a modern society that is tolerant of counter-cultural behaviours).

So the New Age approach does not rule out participation in churches or other forms of traditional religion when these contribute to the individual's self-evaluated well-being. Also, members of traditional religions can, and frequently do, express their individual spiritualities by means of participating in New Age activities outside the specific scope of their religion—for instance reading self-help books, attending personal growth groups, meditating, or decorating their houses (or bodies) in a spiritually-satisfying style.

The specific content of New Age spirituality is almost infinite. The term is usually associated with a somewhat stereotypical interest in esoteric or mystical things such as Zen or Transcendental Medication, occult and paranormal phenomena, or divination techniques such as astrology, Tarot cards and the I Ching. A great deal of the 'self-help' literature can be considered New Age in orientation.

For example, use of acupuncture may go along with Far Eastern interests, or use of herbs or flowers in therapy may mesh with ecological concerns. But almost any object or stimulus might count as New Age healing: what matters is the subjective 'meaning' to the individual—the self-evaluated effect it has on a person's sense of well-being.

The value of healing versus curing

Alternative therapies are often advertised as 'healing', and this word can be interpreted as referring to personal, subjective and psychological benefits. Any specific alternative therapy may or may not benefit any particular individual in this psychological sense. But the range of alternative therapies is very large, and continually growing. Among this vast choice of therapies it is likely that an individual can find some which harmonize with his or her own spiritual goals.

By contrast, orthodox medicine is focused upon curing disease—in which the disease and the cure tend to be defined as objectively and scientifically as possible. The treatment of diabetes focuses on controlling the measured levels of blood sugar, the treatment of pneumonia is focused upon killing the causal germs as detected by laboratory studies. It is naturally desirable that a diabetic or pneumonia patient also be 'healed' in the sense of made to feel subjectively better—but even when this does not happen, the scientific 'cure' is worth having. So, orthodox medicine must cure, and should aim to heal—but does not need to heal; while alternative therapies do not cure—so they must heal in order to be worthwhile.

Because they aim to heal, the explanations of alternative medicine need to have intuitive appeal: they are mythic explanations, not accounts of scientific causality. Myths are stories which function as poetic symbols, and not as literal signs. Myths are meant to imply many things (not just one thing), and have a personal meaning (rather than be an objective description). Scientific theories are not myths—they are intended to be precise descriptions with narrowly-defined meanings.

For example, the meridians of acupuncture have no literal scientific signification. But meridians are suggestive poetic symbols of the way that life can be experienced as a flow of energies, the fact that these energies may come into conflict (yin and yang) and the need for these energies to be balanced. The oriental basis of acupuncture may also appeal, and the precision (and frisson of fear, which must be overcome) of the needle insertion technique may also be intuitively pleasing. If so, then acupuncture might be chosen as one part of a lifestyle.

As another example, perhaps the commonest theme in alternative therapies concerns 'energy'. But this is 'energy' as a positive subjective sense of vitality and harmony—it has nothing to do with the concept of energy as measured by scientific technologies. Indeed, in alternative medicine, the term 'energy' has a multi-faceted, metaphorical quality which stands in stark contrast to the equations of physics.

But another individual may dislike or fail to be engaged by oriental themes, or may find needles too scary, and may instead find a spiritual benefit from contemplating stone age rock carvings or cave paintings. This person might find that healing rituals involving beautiful crystals produce the psychological effects they seek. Healing crystals come with poetic descriptions of the expected effect of each type of crystal, and ways in which they might be deployed to generate these effects.

A person either finds an intuitive plausibility to these descriptions of crystal healing, or they do not. Someone who likes the idea of crystals can try out the rituals, and if this has the desired effect they might continue to do them; but if the rituals don't make the person feel any better, or make them feel worse, then they will presumably give-up crystal healing and might try something else instead — such as aromatherapy, colours, runes, flowers or herbs.

The impossibility of integration

Because New Age healing is based upon individual feelings it is inappropriate (indeed potentially dangerous) when applied to such matters of public policy as science, technology, law, economics — or medicine. But so long as New Age reasoning stays away from these objective areas, its subjective evaluations may have great personal value.

Also, this subjective evaluation system makes New Age healing immune to challenge by science or medicine. New Age validity is a matter of what 'works for me'; contradiction from other people is re-defined as 'your truth'. Individual experience is the ultimate authority, and if an individual claims that they find an alternative therapy to be effective in achieving subjective spiritual goals such as personal harmony and growth, then there can be no argument from medicine or biology. If someone feels energized by an alternative therapy and gains a more positive attitude towards life, then this subjective perception is just as valid as artistic appreciation, preferences among foods or selection of fashions. And the wide range of choice, competition and continual innovation in New Age systems of healing ensures that there is little chance of the public becoming habituated or fatigued by the stimuli on offer — there is always something novel to experience.

New Age spiritualities — including alternative systems of healing — constitute a vast resource of ideas and stimuli, and fulfill a range of useful functions. New Age ideas are published and disseminated widely, for instance in the 'mind, body and spirit' sections of bookshops, in the broadcast mass media and on the Internet. People are free to 'opt-in' to the extent that they find ideas helpful, and are free to ignore anything they do not.

The simultaneous growth of modern medicine and the New Age implies that consumers of alternative healing nearly-always use these therapies broadly appropriately: i.e., for the attainment of subjective personal and spiritual goals, and not for the treatment of diseases. The relationship between orthodox and alternative therapies is therefore potentially a harmonious one.

But clashes are inevitable when both sides claim interpretative authority over the same situation. The major source of conflict is when alternative healing practitioners make claims which purport to be factual but are scientifically incredible. The dilemma is that in the short-term a modicum of science (or pseudo-science) may serve to increase the status of New Age practitioners and validate their activities. Yet, in the longer term, the attempt to subordinate science to spirituality will lead to a conflict which science will win.

Scientists and orthodox physicians who are rightly dismissive of bogus claims to objective effectiveness may in turn deny the subjective benefits of alternative therapies. The situation occurs when medical scientists misunderstand claims of 'healing' as claims of curing disease; or when they try to literalize and ridicule mythic explanations such as the imaginative descriptions of crystal therapy. But this is as misconceived as evaluating the factual accuracy of a poetic metaphor. When Shakespeare asked his mistress: 'Shall I compare thee to a summer's day?', he was not making an equation between the beloved and warm climactic conditions. Contemporary alternative healing is an unstable mixture of science and spirituality. In future it would be better if these incompatible elements would separate out.

The benefits of separation

Alternative medicine will survive and grow most effectively by dropping its scientific pretensions; and becoming candidly mythic, poetic, fictive, symbolic, metaphorical and fantasy-based. This process is already well-advanced in other aspects of New Age spirituality where an explicit appeal to subjective intuition is made.

Orthodox medicine and alternative healing cannot and should not become integrated, for precisely the reason that they are totally different forms of activity with different rules and purposes. To integrate would be to damage what is valuable in each. Randomized trials of New Age therapies are as inappropriate as randomized trials of prayer or the enjoyment of Mozart — such investigations will inevitably be inconclusive, confusing and irrelevant.

As well as there being strong reasons of intellectual principle for separating orthodox and alternative therapies, there are also some strong practical benefits to be gained. In distinction to the graded-education and hierarchical organization of orthodox medicine, alternative therapies typically lack a professional apparatus of training, certification and regulation, and consequently are mostly client-controlled. Another difference is that orthodox medicine is provider-dominated with a narrow range of choice; by contrast, alternative medicine is a marketplace offering a vast and growing range of choices. Orthodox medicine resembles a highly restricted but nutritionally-balanced diet; alternative therapies are like an endless pick-and-mix banquet from which the consumer selects what they fancy, taste it, then decide whether to eat more or try something else.

New Age healing deploys the placebo effect and the personality of the therapist in a much freer and more powerful way than can be achieved in orthodox medicine. Alternative healers will be impaired if required to work within strict theoretical and organizational confines. When healing depends on therapeutic charisma, professional and standardized forms of education and accreditation will just tend to weed-out some of the most potentially helpful personalities.

Alternative medicine fits very well with some of the dominant attributes of modern society because it is characterized by continual generation of choice and depends upon the mass media for dissemination of information. Clients hear about alternative therapies from newspapers, magazines, television, the internet; and by advertising. Their knowledge of the explanations and theories of alternative healing comes from media stories, product labels, and whatever a therapist tells them in private. The bulk of alternative therapy is self-administered — people buy products, enjoy the explanations, read the instructions, and treat themselves.

In situations where clients consult with alternative therapists, it is likely that the role of charisma has a vital part to play. A popular therapist will probably have a 'therapeutic personality' such that personal interaction makes most clients feel better. But personality clashes are inevitable, even for a highly charismatic healer, which is why wide choice and client-control of the consultation is of such great importance in alternative therapy.

In orthodox medicine things are different. A physician may try to present the standard scientific explanation underlying therapy in an intuitively-appealing way — but even if this attempt fails, the treatment should still be useful since its effectiveness has typically been objectively evaluated. Surgery or chemotherapy may make the patient feel much worse in the short term, even when they succeed in curing cancer. Of course, it is a great advantage if orthodox medicine is practiced by charismatic doctors. But with orthodox medicine, charisma is an optional extra: the medicine will still work in its absence.

But there are no objective boundaries on the explanations offered by alternative therapists, or provided with New Age products, because clients vary so widely in what they find convincing. In alternative healing, the explanation must be intuitively-appealing to the client, here-and-now, or else the therapy will not succeed in making the client feel better. Indeed, so long as the therapy does no significant harm, intuitive benefit is the beginning and end of evaluation in alternative medicine.

Conclusion

I envisage a future in which orthodox and alternative therapies both thrive, but separately. Orthodox medicine is based on scientific theories and is characterized by objective evaluation criteria and formal professional structures of education and certification. In contrast, alternative healing deploys a wide range of intuitively-appealing but non-scientific explanations, and constitutes a consumer-dominated marketplace of ideas and therapies which are personally-evaluated by the client.

Orthodox medicine focuses on curing disease and promoting health. But alternative therapies should instead be focused on promoting well-being and personal fulfillment. To accomplish this, alternative therapists need to be able freely to deploy personal charisma and richly mythic explanations. In conclusion, alternative therapies are neither medical nor scientific, but they should be respected as a potential contribution to modern spiritual well-being.

Asbjørn Hróbjartsson

Research on Complementary or Alternative Medicine

The importance and frailty of impartiality

People make research

The first complementary-alternative medicine conference I attended was a lively affair with participants from several continents. The researchers walked around from one lecture hall to another, all with their identical conference bags. Often two middle-aged persons would stop, smile, pat each other on the shoulder, talk for a while and then rush on. I was flabbergasted by the show, and remember standing in a corner, looking around, and feeling the loneliness that comes with doing research, and with which I had been struggling, slowly evaporate.

During the conference I saw the real experts, the men and women whose names and work I was intimately familiar with, but whom I did not know personally. I had spent a couple of years meticulously studying the most important research papers of a field closely related to complementary-alternative medicine. For me, these papers became mental cornerstones, small but important points of solidity, the place where doubt became meaningless. I trusted these papers.

So, to meet some of the people behind the papers was fascinating. I realised that the papers that I had read, and so admired, and so trusted, were other persons' brainchildren. Names became faces. It suddenly struck me, banal as it may be, that persons make research. I was slightly troubled by this. Some of the faces belonged to friendly persons, some not, some were charming, and some not. In many ways, beside a telling intelligence and persistence, they resembled most persons, persons with ideologies, idiosyncrasies, and particular points of views.

Later that conference I told an older colleague of my uneasiness. His reply was cynical: 'We all know corners are cut. Some researchers have integrity and some not. The main reason I go to scientific conferences is not to listen to the talks and get information on the newest research, but to meet the guys, look them in the eyes, to figure out who writes a paper I can trust.'

Researchers make mistakes

To take a conclusion from a medical research paper at face value you need to trust. You need to trust several persons on several levels. You need to trust the good intentions of the persons who conducted the research, that the methods they used were appropriate, and that the methods were carried out correctly.

However, research methods are complicated. Researchers make mistakes. Errors in medical research are frequent, both in the sense of inappropriate methods, and incorrect implementation of otherwise appropriate methods. Doug Altman, a leading medical statistician and research methodologist, forcefully and aptly described this: 'The scandal of poor medical research' (Altman, 1994).

By carefully studying a research article it is sometimes possible to decide whether to trust the appropriateness of the methods. However, it is much more difficult to decide whether to trust the good intentions of the researchers. Readers of research papers are kind and tend to assume the good intentions of the persons behind the research. In general, such a trust may be somewhat casual, but in the case of complementary-alternative medicine it is naïve.

The main question I raise in this essay is: 'What is the role of impartiality in research on complementary-alternative research?' My thesis is that research on complementary-alternative medicine is conducted in a setting of strong tension between groups of persons with hard held views, and that this tension threatens the reliability of research results.

Methods matter

Research on complementary-alternative medicine is broad, span-
ning from case stories of individual patients, laboratory studies, to
epidemiological studies, just to mention a few fields. For reasons of
clarity many of the examples and issues discussed below concern
one type of research, randomised clinical trials, but in most cases the
problems raised will have general implication for empirical research
on complementary-alternative medicine.

It is fruitful to focus on randomised clinical trials. First, the randomised clinical trial is the most reliable method of evaluating the
effect of an intervention, and the question of the possible effects of
complementary and alternative interventions is at the forefront of
the debate. Second, there has been considerable attention on the
methodological quality of trials and we know at least some of the
characteristics of a reliable trial.

In principle, a randomised trial is a clinical experiment in which
patients are allocated to a control group and an experimental group.
The control group receives the control intervention, for example a
placebo. The experimental group receives the experimental intervention, for example a drug. The unique aspect of a randomised trial
is that the two groups of patients are comparable, at least as long as
the randomisation is conducted correctly, and the trial is fairly large.
So, in theory, if significantly more patients in the experimental
group improve during the trial, compared with the control group,
we can be fairly certain that the intervention works.

What characterises a well-performed trial? One important aspect
is how the randomisation of patients is performed. It is crucial that
the person who enrols patients into the trial, and allocates them to
the experimental or the control group, is unaware of what type of
treatment the forthcoming patient is supposed to get. This is the case
if the doctor telephones a special centralised randomisation unit that
irreversibly enrols a patient before disclosing the allocated
treatment.

Also, blinding patients minimises biased reporting of symptoms,
and blinding data collectors minimise biased interpretation of clinical signs. Furthermore, low drop-out rates are preferable. Of course,
other aspects are important too, for example the size of the trial, the
statistical analysis, and the type of funding.

Editors of scientific journals struggle with how to separate reliable
trials from unreliable trials. Many editors use peer reviewers. Peers
of the authors of a submitted trial report review it, and give sugges-

tions for changes and recommendations for rejection or publication. A major issue for peer reviewer recommendations is whether the methods used are regarded appropriate.

Further empirical methodological studies will hopefully widen our knowledge of the relative importance of each methodological quality factor, and identify other factors.[1] But at the end of the day, regardless of how many methodological factors we add to the list, we end up facing the problem that reliable and adequate methods are only reliable and adequate if performed by researchers who are dedicated to these methods, who take them seriously, and not just go through the motions. In other words, methods matter, but so do researchers.

Researchers matter

It is unlikely to find a chapter on researcher partiality in a textbook on trial methodology, and many researchers and commentators tend to shy from the problem, maybe because they feel uncomfortable by openly discussing a subjective aspect of research. However, the issue has been faced directly by the International Committee of Medical Journal Editors (the so-called 'Vancouver Group'). They require that authors of research papers declare so-called 'conflicts of interest'.

Conflicts of interests are often thought of as financial. Many trials are sponsored by a pharmaceutical or device company, and several authors of trial reports are on the advisory board of such companies, own stocks, or have received money for giving talks or advice. In addition, company employees frequently initiate the trial, write the protocol, do the statistical analysis, and write up a first draft of the trial report. Finally, often the 'academic' authors of the subsequently published trial paper are restricted in their academic freedom through written contracts enabling the companies to suppress publication of what they regard as problematic information that could influence sales (Gøtzsche *et al.*, 2006.) Positive conclusions are found more often in industry funded trials than non-industry funded trials (and this tendency is independent of the reported results) (Als-Nielsen *et al.*, 2003).

Companies or individuals produce complementary-alternative medicine for profit, for example Chinese herbs, homeopathic preparations, Ginseng, vitamin and minerals. There is little reason to

---

[1] See http://www.icmje.org

believe that the producers of complementary-alternative medicines and devices are less biased than other pharmacological and device companies. In some cases herbs have been adulterated with conventional drugs, for example corticosteroids (Ernst, 2002).

However, the medical journal editors of the Vancouver Group also emphasise that conflicts of interest can be 'academic competition, and intellectual passion'.[2] A dedicated and original researcher needs passion for his or her topic; however, the demands of competition in research for fame and positions may cause a conflict with good research practice. Similarly, when two groups of researchers disagree passionately, it may be challenging to interpret fairly a research result that favours the opposing group's position. The creative passion for a research topic is different from the more precarious passion for a specific research result.

What the editors acknowledge is that good research is conducted by researchers with a high degree of impartiality. Impartiality is generally understood as a sense of fairness, neutrality, independence, or objectivity. An impartial trial researcher is one with a genuine interest in finding out whether or not the intervention is effective. He or she is impartial to the intervention tested, or to any competing intervention, or to any financial or ideological implication of a certain research result.

Strictly speaking, impartiality means that the researchers have no preference whatsoever for either the compared treatments. In reality most researchers will have some inclination to one of them, likely more often to the experimental than to the control treatment. If this inclination is mild it may not cause a problem, as there is still substantial doubt as to which treatment is regarded the most effective. Furthermore, some researchers are probably able to contain considerable personal preferences for a treatment, or strong religious or other convictions, from their research. Still, it is difficult to know when containment is successful, and it is reasonable to assume that the risk of bias increases with the degree of partiality.

The bias associated with strong partiality may be unintentional and involve many decisions during the planning, the execution, the data handling, and the writing of the manuscript, that require a substantial degree of subjective judgement. However, the bias can also be conscious. Modifications to a trial's design can be made so to produce favourable results, for example, outcomes that are statistically significant can be selected for publication (and as primary out-

[2]   http://www.icmje.org

comes), thus suppressing negative findings, and giving a biased picture of the effect of the intervention (Chan *et al.*, 2004). The most extreme example of strong researcher partiality is fraud involving fabrication of data. Though difficult to assess, such data fabrication is hopefully rare but high profile cases continue to be exposed (*Lancet*, 2006).

Research results and hard-held views

The ideal of the impartial researcher sometimes meets with considerable pressure from views that originate from religious, ideological, or political convictions. One historic example of the clash between research and religion concerns the former medical student Galileo, who in 1632, a long time after turning to mathematics and physics, published the book *Dialogue on the Two Chief World Systems*. Here he argued that the earth circled around the sun. For this he was charged with heresy by the inquisition, and at the age of seventy, forced to renounce his views. Legend has it that when he rose from his knees after his renouncement, he whispered – 'And yet it moves' (referring to earth). However, the execution of Giordano Bruno, burned in 1600 for similar views, would have made such a whisper perilous.

The fate of Giordano Bruno and Galileo is often told as a chilling tale of the dogmatism of the dark ages, and by implication, as a comforting story of the enlightened society of today. The movement of planets causes no controversy in the twenty-first century, and at least in democracies, governments do not persecute scientists with unpopular views. Research is held in high esteem, and scientific results accumulate to the better of mankind. We would like to think that if a tension develops between research and religion, or another hard-held view, such a tension is of small significance and of limited duration, as research will quickly prevail over dogma. However, the tensions between research and hard-held views, full-blown and brutal in the historical case of Galileo, still exist, but in a more contained and moderate form.

Think of areas like body-mind interaction, gender, race, ecology, processed food production, homosexuality, HIV prevention, abortion, or stem cell research. Or think of questions like 'Are homosexual couples better or worse parents than heterosexual couples?', 'Is advising sexual abstinence more or less effective than condoms in preventing HIV?', 'Can negative thinking cause heart attacks?', 'Do blacks have higher or lower intelligence than Asians?', 'Is eating ecologically grown cereals good or bad for your health?', 'Do artificial sweeteners cause cancer?' or 'When does a foetus feel pain?'.

These research questions repeatedly cause controversy. Strong feelings are provoked, headlines made. The point here is not who is right, but that research on these topics is conducted in an environment of strong ideological positions, of hard held views.

Complementary-alternative medicine and hard-held views

Complementary-alternative medicine is another example of a highly controversial research topic. Even giving a description of what characterises complementary-alternative medicine may be controversial. The following description follow the outlines presented by Kaptchuk, trained in oriental medicine, and Miller, a medical ethicist (Kaptchuk and Miller, 2005). Complementary -alternative medicine (for example acupuncture, homeopathy, Chinese herbal medicine, crystal therapy, reflexology, psychic clairvoyance) represents a heterogeneous group of theoretical backgrounds and interventions, but there are some common traits. First, many types of complementary-alternative interventions have theoretical backgrounds that originate from a revered authoritative figure or text (e.g. Samuel Hahnemann for homeopathy, or the Yellow Emperor's Classic of Internal Medicine for East Asian Medicine). Second, the theory is (apparently) incongruent with established physical, chemical and biological science. Third, any changes to the theoretical corpus and practices are based on authoritative figures that reinterpret the established theory in light of accumulated experience. Fourth, the interventions are mostly validated by ordinary human experience, for example single case stories of 'unimpeachable testimonials', or the intuition of the practitioners.

Complementary-alternative medicine provokes strong feelings. Somewhat simplified, there are the believers and the sceptics. In short, believers in complementary-alternative are in opposition to the power structures of the medical establishment. Mainstream medicine is regarded as narrowly mechanistic, simplistically rational, and pharmaceutically dominated. It is seen as a form of medicine that has lost sight of the feelings and spirituality of the individual patient in a cold maze of big careers, big bucks, statistics and laboratory tubes. In short, the believers regard mainstream medicine as dehumanised conservatism.

The sceptics, on the other hand, see complementary-alternative medicine as a backlash into an unscientific way of thinking. They regard alternative-complementary medicine as an irrational and romantic movement that deludes itself, and its patients, by caring more about simplistic, but superficially meaningful, explanations to complex problems, than about distinguishing proven facts from speculative ideas. Similarly, the lack of an ideal of experimentally testing the beneficial and harmful effect of interventions is regarded as hazardous. In short, the sceptics regard complementary-alternative medicine as quasi-religious dogmatism.

It is no surprise that believers and sceptics tend to conflict, sometimes quite intensely. The conflict has the character of an ideological clash. Still, for quite different reasons a strict believer in complementary-alternative medicine and a strict sceptic will tend to agree that research into complementary-alternative medicine is not worthwhile, or even absurd. The strict believer is convinced that the interventions work; the strict sceptic is convinced that the interventions do not work. Strict believers and sceptics do not tend to conduct trials. Their strong partiality is, however, of relevance when the results of trials run by others are discussed and interpreted (Hróbjartsson and Brorson, 2002).

At times, strict believers and sceptics are involved in randomised clinical trials on complementary-alternative medicine for opportunistic reasons. Some sceptics want to prove (what they already think they know) that there is no effect of an intervention. Similarly, some believers want to prove (what they already think they know) that there is an effect. Commonly, such strict sceptics and believers are interested in proving whether complementary-alternative medicine as such 'is true or not' (and not the effect of a specific treatment). However, randomised trials cannot stand alone in such global assessments that also involve results from other types of research, value judgement and common sense. In any case, trials conducted by persons with strong partiality have a considerable risk of biased conclusions.

However, some moderate believers are in doubt. They may find it problematic that frequently used interventions have not been tested for beneficial and harmful effects, and that when randomised trials of complementary-alternative interventions are conducted they mostly find little evidence of an effect. Similarly, some moderate sceptics, as myself, are in doubt. We may find it puzzling that complementary-alternative medicine is so popular, and acknowledge that effective interventions could have been developed by accident, intuition or experience, or that the patient-provider interaction could be associated with effects. Thus, despite quite substantial dis-agreements and a tendency for ideologically based hostility, it should sometimes be possible to fulfil one of the characteristics of good research: that impartial persons perform the research.

The lack of a research tradition within complementary-alternative medicine causes problems for those who want to conduct random-ised trials. First, many believers in complementary-alternative med-icine are inexperienced with clinical trial methodology, and will often have to learn them as they go along, with a risk of conducting trials with sub-optimal methods. Second, many sceptics that engage in randomised clinical trials may have a knowledge of research methodology, but will generally not have an intimate knowledge of the practices of complementary-alternative medicine, and if they are not able to acquire the necessary skills and knowledge, risk con-ducting trials that are clinically irrelevant.

Maybe the most serious consequence of a lack of research tradition is that the ethos of research is difficult to acquire. The ethos of research goes beyond just being in doubt about the effect of an inter-vention, it implies an abstract critical and self-critical way of think-ing, in which established knowledge is regarded fallible and modifiable by reason and structured observation, and it involves taking a pride in the careful execution of good methodological stan-dards. It is often acquired in a kind of apprentice relation between a young and an experienced researcher. To fully incorporate this way of thinking may also be a considerable challenge for a moderate believer in complementary-alternative medicine.

What can be done about partiality in research on complementary-alternative medicine? First, I think a change of perspective is needed. We should stop avoiding the problem, and start con-sciously and openly addressing partiality. Thus, when appraising the risk of bias in research it is insufficient to look only at the appro-priateness of the methods used. A fuller picture involves the abstract, but nonetheless essential, personal aspect of research: the commitment of the researcher to do an impartial exploration. A chal-lenge to this process is to assess when there is a case of harmless minor partiality and when there is a case of considerable partiality with substantial risk of bias.

Second, we need pragmatic tools to identify and handle partiality in research. A formal declaration of impartiality is difficult to imple-ment without clear criteria, may be seen as overly formal, and will not identify the researchers that do not comply. However, sometimes an informal declaration can be deduced from the text of a research paper. Collaborative trial research groups could be formed that include both sceptics and believers. Furthermore, when interpreting trial results it seems rational to trust the believers' trials more when they find no effects, and to trust the sceptics' trials more when they find an effect. At this point we may only scratch the surface, but an increased awareness of the problem of partiality in research on complementary-alternative medicine is a necessary starting point for further discussion.

Complementary-alternative medicine and the randomised clinical trial

Strict believers in complementary-alternative medicine tend to regard randomised clinical trials unsuited for testing the effects of complementary-alternative interventions because these are regarded as uniquely different from other types of interventions. The randomised trial is seen as 'the method of mainstream medicine'.

Interestingly, several of the first trials using the principle of randomisation were conducted within complementary-alternative medicine, for example in telepathy in 1884 (Richet, 1884). In medicine the first truly randomised trial was only conducted in 1948, and it took 15–25 years of intense methodological discussion before the medical research community reached a reasonable degree of consensus that the randomised trial was more reliable in assessing effect, than other methods. There continues to be an ongoing discussion of the possible bias involved in randomised trials.

In my view, the awareness of the gross errors involved in other types of evaluations of therapeutic interventions, and the subsequent development and implementation of the randomised trial is one of the most important developments of medical knowledge. Still, standard medical research methods have progressed over time. From a philosophical point of view it is conceivable that well performed methodological research at some point in the future could identify other types of evaluation methods that in certain situations are more reliable than the randomised trial. However, it is also conceivable that methodological research cannot identify such methods. The point here is that the question is not solved by assumptions, or ideologically based dogma, but by further research by methodologists using rational arguments and empirical observations. Impartiality of the methodological researchers is just as important as the impartiality of other types of researchers.

Conclusion

The role of impartiality in research on complementary-alternative medicine is one of importance and frailty. Impartiality is important because research conducted by partial researchers has a considerable risk of biased conclusions. Impartiality is frail because research on complementary-alternative medicine is conducted in a setting of strong ideologically based tension between believers and sceptics. Lack of impartiality threatens the reliability of research on complementary-alternative medicine.

References

Als-Nielsen, B., Chen, W., Gluud, C., Kjaergard, L.L. (2003), 'Association of funding and conclusions in randomized drug trials: a reflection of treatment effect or adverse events?', *Journal of the American Medical Association* (JAMA), 290:7, 921-8.

Altman, D.G. (1994), 'The scandal of poor medical research', in *British Medical Journal*, 308, 283-4.

Chan, A.W., Hróbjartsson, A., Haahr, M.T., Gøtzsche, P.C., Altman, D.G. (2004), 'Empirical evidence for selective reporting of outcomes in randomized trials: Comparison of protocols to publications', in JAMA, 291, 2457-65

Ernst, E. (2002), 'Adulteration of Chinese herbal medicines with synthetic drugs: a systematic review', in *Journal of International Medicine*, 252:2, 107-13. Review.

Gøtzsche, P.C., Hróbjartsson, A., Johansen, H.K., Haahr, M.T., Altman, D.G., Chan, A.W. (2006), 'Restrictions on academic freedom in industry-initiated randomised clinical trials', in JAMA, 295:14, 1645-6.

Hróbjartsson, A., Brorson, S. (2002), 'Interpreting results from randomized clinical trials of complementary / alternative interventions: the role of trial quality and pre-trial beliefs, I', in *The Role of Complementary and Alternative Medicine, Accomodating Pluralism*, ed. D. Callahan (Washington DC: Georgetown University Press), 107-21.

Kaptchuk, T.J. and Miller, F.G. (2005), 'Viewpoint: what is the best and most ethical model for the relationship between mainstream and alternative medicine: opposition, integration, or pluralism?', in *Academic Medicine*, 80:3, 286-90.

Lancet (2006). Editorial. 'Writing a new ending for a story of scientific fraud', in *Lancet* 367:1, 9504.

Richet, C. (1884), 'La suggestion mentale et le calcule des probabilités', in *Revue Philosophique de la France et de l'Étranger*, 18, 609-74.

James Randi

An Amateur's View of the CAM Scene

At the outset, let me make one thing perfectly clear: my qualifications concerning this subject, alternative/complementary medicine, here referred to as 'CAM', consist mostly of common sense, a wide-ranging experience of flimflam, and extensive exposure to a great variety of scam artists. Those rascals have discovered that a large percentage of the population will react to almost anything presented from a position of authority—particularly if the name of the presenter bears the magical letters, 'PhD'. I have long maintained that an education only makes you educated, and that it takes much more than that, to make you smart; experience of the outside world is required. Please have no doubts at all about my strong respect for formal education, but I've found that many highly educated persons simply don't think clearly in the real world that I inhabit. I don't have the privilege of appending letters to my name, though no less an authority than Isaac Asimov once generously commented that I had a very good grasp of the scientific method despite my lack of any advanced formal education. One of my thoroughly lettered detractors in the UK, speaking before the Royal Society some years ago, referred to me as a 'mere conjuror'; in response to that designation I told him, 'Conjuror, yes, but "mere" —*never!*'

I regret to say that much of the blame for unfounded belief in outlandish modes of medical care must be laid at the doorstep of academia. The plain fact is that the public is largely ignorant of what science is all about. They picture men—women less frequently—dressed in white coats scurrying about bearing mysterious smoking test tubes. And, they tend to fear and reject that which they don't understand. They do, however, tend to pay attention to statements that bear the imprimatur of scientists. Thus, when those scientists fail to provide proper information, they fail their public.

Examples of misbehaviour

Even within recent years, we've had many startling examples of scientists who have betrayed their positions. A 2001 study from Columbia University Medical School published in the respected, peer-reviewed *Journal of Reproductive Medicine*, reported that in-vitro fertilization was twice as likely to result in pregnancy if patients were prayed for by total strangers halfway around the world — without the knowledge of the patients. Now, if that were true, it would certainly be a revolutionary discovery. However, it turned out that most of that data was simply invented to prove a favoured point of view. After being alerted to look more closely into the reports, the lead author of the paper resigned. Another of the paper's authors — a known con-artist named Daniel Wirth, though known under many aliases — is presently still in prison for this and other offences. Amazingly, to this day, six years since the hoax was revealed, neither Columbia University nor the *Journal of Reproductive Medicine* has chosen to withdrawn this bogus paper; they have ignored all pressure from the academic world, and are to be found in residence in a local Ivory Tower. Indeed, the most recent declaration from Editor-in-Chief Lawrence D. Devoe, M.D. of the *Journal of Reproductive Medicine*, repeats that he will not withdraw the article, and Columbia University ignores all requests to act on the matter.[1]

In 2002, Dr Jan Hendrik Schön of Bell Labs announced in *Nature* magazine that he had produced a bio-derived transistor on the molecular scale, a claim which if true would have overturned the silicon-based electronics industry. It was a lie, a total invention. Bell Labs fired Schön, and nineteen of his already-published scientific papers were withdrawn, along with his academic degree.

In 2004, the exciting and revolutionary cloning/stem cell work announced by Dr Woo Suk Hwang at Seoul National University — once widely acclaimed — was found to be spurious. The journal *Science*, which had innocently published his work, immediately retracted both his papers — without even turning to glance in the direction of any Ivory Tower for refuge.

In all of these matters, it was suggested by observing academics that the scientists' fellow workers might not have been sufficiently critical of the claimed findings and/or procedures, in view of their exceptional nature. Had any of them exercised sufficient professional responsibility in examining the integrity of the presented

[1]   Details on the matter can be found at
      http://www.randi.org/jr/121704no.html#2

data, the reputation of science as a sometimes mad house, might have been avoided. I daresay that Marie Curie's work — revolutionary as it was — was profoundly vetted.

The unsinkable rubber ducks

In my work as an investigator of highly unusual claims, I find that there seems to be no limit to what will be accepted and even embraced by the 'true believer'. This is particularly evident in the field of CAM. It's no surprise at all that the public is more interested in bogus medical claims than in claims of perpetual motion, speaking with the dead, or yogic levitation; they can entertain those subjects in more detail after they get to feel better.

The quacks adopt protective coloration, as nature would incline them to do; they insist that what they're doing is a 'science', though often even the term 'pseudoscience' would not encompass their philosophies. What they call 'research' is usually nothing more than amassing anecdotal material, that by sheer volume can impress the naïve, and they have enthusiastically embraced the currently popular practice of 'meta-analysis', in which huge amounts of data are evaluated and summed up in a search for significance that — if it can barely make that hurdle — will be celebrated in the media. What's not properly taken into account is that word 'evaluated', the factor upon which the strength of the entire procedure depends; if any data is over-valued, the results can be fatally skewed, and the experimenters themselves usually do the evaluation of the power of the data-sets. In practice, it's common to find that they have diligently searched the available literature for any pale ghost of a suggestion or a hint that can be applied to apparently validate their claims. They will pester any number of academics until they find one with a pathologically-significant Achilles Heel, one who will accede to their needs and perhaps even issue a statement to that effect. Even a cursory examination of the qualifications of such endorsers often reveals their previous acceptance of quack notions, thus illuminating their actual authority.

It is quite true that CAM practitioners often offer not only treatment for specific medical problems, but a realignment of everything from domestic relationships to financial outlooks — thus a return to the personalized patient/physician connection which a generation ago seemed to have vanished. The phenomenon of a bedside visit may not be experienced again, but in my opinion, it needs to return.

Personally, I have a problem with the attitude of many scientists, those who seem to believe that they are not subject to the rules of reality. Many of those who consider themselves scientists have no problem flying in the face of reason if their formal work conforms to the cosmetic criteria that will make it acceptable to their peers; to them, form is everything. Copious references, the proper catchwords, and a raft of footnotes often seem to do the job in that respect. The only other field that outdoes this for pretension, is the murky one of patent application; there, anyone can easily get lost in obfuscation, and subsequently just about any fanciful notion can be issued a patent number. Just recently, for example, the peanut-butter-and-jelly sandwich was patented — U.S. Patent # 6,004,596 …

Examples of obvious flummery

I admit that in discussing the field of CAM I am primarily concerned with homeopathy, largely because of the enormous impact that this particular form of popular quackery is having on the whole area of medical care. While the use of magnets applied to the body, the invocation of mystical 'vibrations', and the chanting of sacred sounds — all part of so much of the CAM landscape — must also be handled, I'll deal here with such matters relatively briefly.

The famous Florsheim Shoe Company has now been supplying the American public with high-quality footwear for 115 years. Then, in 1998, they introduced the 'MagneForce' shoe as the 'first shoe with its own power supply'. Yes, the mind boggles at such language, and at such a concept, but there was much more to this. There were tiny magnets imbedded in the soles of these special shoes, at a cost of an extra $25 to the buyer. Florsheim — through one Gary Null, their resident PhD who'd obtained his degree by mail-order — claimed that such a magnetic field applied to the body would stimulate blood circulation and had been shown to reduce pain and to increase 'natural' healing. They touted the 'rapid healing and relief' produced, and 'reduction in foot, leg and back fatigue, an increase in the range of motion, reduced leg, hip and back pain, and resulting greater energy levels' from the MagneForce product. They claimed that 'numerous clinical tests conducted at such institutions as Vanderbilt University, New York University and Baylor University have documented' these advantages, and that diabetics could thereby benefit, as well.

What's more, these weren't just ordinary magnets concealed in the shoes; the literature issued by Florsheim revealed that they were 'unipolar' magnets! Though such a magnet does not and cannot exist, the inevitable Nobel Prize that immediately appears within grasp upon such a development, let alone the major revolution in technology and basic physics, need not be mentioned. Moreover, 'Dr' Null endorses the use of magnets and laetrile for curing cancer, he opposes vaccination, recommends coffee enemas, and declares that 'misaligned' bony plates of the skull cause a raft of medical problems—all notions that have been shown quite erroneous. Still, Null is regularly featured by PBS-TV during fund-raising campaigns, because quackery sells to the naïve. Another howler by Null was published in the small book that accompanied the Florsheim wonder-shoes: 'The earth [sic] itself is a giant magnet, with north and south poles and a hot liquid core. The hot liquid core creates a magnetic field which at the earth's [sic] surface is relatively weak, but serves to keep humans attached to the earth [sic]. Without this magnetic field, we would spin into outer space.'

Reading this incredible statement, I commented that it might be true if we wore manhole-covers on each foot, though that would seriously inhibit clog-dancing and swimming.

We see countless devices openly sold by such leading merchants as the Walgreen Pharmacies in the USA and by Boots in the UK, offering everything from sleep-shades to dog beds with the added feature of imbedded plastic magnets. As Bob Park of the American Physical Association has deftly pointed out, magnetic fields put out by strapped-on bits of refrigerator-ad composition magnets are not only obviously too weak to have any discernible effect—biological or otherwise—but the magnetic field present is directed in a tight pattern that lies essentially within the device itself.

As for the matter of 'vibrations', a word almost inevitably introduced in texts touting pseudoscience, those who invoke such phenomena would not recognize them if presented with a basket full. The term is thrown about as if it were a magical phenomenon. Electromagnetic, auditory, or hand-delivered vibrations are simply the result of an oscillation back-and-forth on either side of a neutral point. They can be observed on a clock pendulum, a tuning fork, or a backyard wash line in a brisk wind. Nothing mysterious at all, a perfectly natural phenomenon. And, freely teamed up with the vibrations are 'quantum' phenomena, a term invoked to further obfuscate.

The major villain

Homeopathy is the use of medicinal substances so diluted that effectively zero concentrations are achieved, depending upon definitions of purity and significance levels. The usual dilutions in homeopathy are beyond Avogadro's number, which I prefer to express in the long form, as 1 part of medicament in 602,252,000,000,000,000,000,000,000 parts of diluent—to make more evident to my audiences just how ridiculous the claims of efficacy are. Most packaging of these sham medicines proudly assure the potential user that there will be 'no side effects'. What they fail to add, is that there will be no effect at all—except to relieve that ugly lump in your wallet.

Homeopathy thus meets the definition of magic, in that it purports to produce its effects through mysterious influences—'vibrations' or 'memory'—that are, by all known rules and laws of the universe, beyond possibility. Of course, from my pragmatic, rational, point of view, I would require only one example of the proof of this strange claim, to evaporate that statement. Homeopathy has a basic appeal because it involves a very fundamental substance—water, one of the basic requirements and building-blocks of life as we know it. This is an attractive, simplistic, and beguiling scenario to those who can dispense with actual evidence and rely on anecdotal material for assurance.

To illustrate the way that merchandisers have taken advantage of the naïvety of the consumer, consider the case of Zicam—an immensely popular treatment for the symptoms of colds in the USA. This is one of small group of remedies that chooses to label itself as 'homeopathic', but actually contains ingredients in measurable and medically-effective amounts. This is clear evidence of the attraction of quackery to the uninformed. Such products—generally speaking—cost forty to seventy per cent more than products that are actually active, and since Zicam demonstrably works and is—falsely—believed to be homeopathic in nature, the actual homeopathic industry is thus made far more acceptable to consumers.

Enter Benveniste

One of the most prominent modern academics to support the claims of homeopathy was Dr Jacques Benveniste (1935-2004) with whom I had more than a decade of discussion on the subject. In a bitter and disinformative article in the Spring/1998 issue of *The Anomalist* titled 'On the role of stage magicians in biological research', Benveniste mockingly referred to my actual, practical, involvement in science as limited to once being 'A scientist; a real live laboratory technician!' He was thereby—quite correctly—warning his (and my) readers that I was an unlettered commentator on the subject he held dearest. He never examined the possibility that I might have known what I was talking about.

The most evident problem for scientists who have chosen to bypass orthodox standards of their trade, as Benveniste did, is that when double-blind methods have been applied to CAM procedures and regimens, they have largely failed to produce positive results; homeopathy is one such subject. Indeed, arguments are offered to the effect that regular scientific procedures — and particularly double-blind provisions — should not or can not be applied to the testing of CAM claims. One prominent authority on homeopathic practice — Alexandra Delinick, M.D. — says clearly that 'Homeopathy, its philosophy and remedies, is clearly a science that can not be relegated to the existing reductionist philosophy and present scientific paradigm' (Delinick, 0000). This is in effect saying that this facet of CAM is in a special 'magical' category that takes it out of the consideration of science and reason. This blatant contradiction seems to have no significance for those scientists who endorse the use of homeopathy. Indeed, when Brian Josephson — the British Nobel Laureate, and an enthusiastic supporter of the practice of homeopathy — taunted the American Physical Society, challenging them to test the results claimed by homeopath Jacques Benveniste, he apparently was shocked by the fact that the APS not only promptly accepted, but offered to pay all costs of what would obviously be an expensive and thorough experiment. I of course also agreed to put my foundation's million-dollar prize into the pot, but to no avail; we not only never heard another word from Josephson nor from Benveniste, but they cut off all correspondence with the APS and with me, and *never returned to the discussion*. Strange.

When it comes to making excuses, a frequently-invoked 'out' is that homeopathic remedies have been tested using animals such as horses, as subjects. It is argued that animals cannot lie, cannot be influenced by the placebo effect, and are effectively 'blank slates' for the production of definitive data; included in that argument is the gleeful declaration that double-blind provisions for such tests are therefore unnecessary. The obvious fact is that, since horses also cannot be expected to answer surveys or give personal opinions or reports on their medical conditions, those answers must be sought from the owners and handlers of the animals. These people can be expected to be sympathetic to positive results from homeopathy, since they've given permission to use their animals and their facilities for such a test. Of course, this difficulty could be avoided simply by not informing anyone but the randomizers involved in the double-blind test, which supplied medications were, and were not, supposedly active substances, and which were 'controls'. This was not the kind of test that has been used when animals are involved, which means that these tests, too, are invalid and useless.

What's actually in there?

But what are the actual 'ingredients' in homeopathic preparations? This, as I found out when I addressed members of the European Union in Oslo some years ago on the subject, is quite a surprise to anyone who has not actually looked into the matter. I hold in my hand a package of homeopathic medicine labeled, 'Insomnia'. It also states that it's a 'New Superior Formula' at a 'Triple Level Potency'. On the back of the container I see a list of the ingredients, the major one of which is '*Coffea Cruda 7x, 9x, & 12x*.' This translates as one part in 10 million, one part in 1000 million, and one part in one million, million, of coffee bean content. Note, please, that the actual ingredient is a coffee bean, not even instant coffee extract. Knowing how many coffee beans are required to brew a cup of coffee, this reduces *ad absurdum* any notion that caffeine could be detected—by any means, chemical, spectroscopic, or dowsing rod. Perhaps you didn't notice, I must point out that the use of coffee to defeat insomnia is quite in line with homeopathic practice. Is it now becoming evident that the more one understands about homeopathy, the less rational and believable its claims become?

In preparing a text for use in a book which will have highly experienced and qualified contributors, one runs the risk of repetition of previously-handled situations. I trust that my amateur efforts may have given the reader a slightly different approach to quackery and irrationality. Just because a particular facet of the quackery industry has not been mentioned above, please do not assume that it's outside of my scope; there is a wide spectrum of nonsense, both medical and scientific, that I handle every day. I refer you to our webpage at www.randi.org to examine the plethora of wild and unproven claims that we deal with. In closing, I must tell you that several acquaintances have described my work as being anti-Darwinian, in that it interferes with the natural selection process with which we are so familiar. I will leave you to ponder on that matter.

References

Benveniste, J. (1998), 'On the role of stage magicians in biological research', in *The Anomalist*.

John Garrow

CAM in Court

Honest trading

Any civilisation that engages in trading needs a system that assures the purchaser that what he buys is genuine. Throughout recorded history, rulers have issued currency stamped so that the value of each coin is identified and guaranteed, and their officers have punished traders who traded in counterfeit money or goods. Today we have a Trade Descriptions Act (TDA) that is widely applied. This Act requires that any descriptions of goods or services, given by a person acting in the course of a trade or business, should be accurate and not misleading. For example a publican who charges for a pint of beer, or a shot of Gordon's gin, but who dispenses a different volume of beer, or a different type of gin, risks prosecution under the TDA.

The same principle that regulates publicans applies to those offering goods or services in the field of healthcare. For example, if an advertiser claims that a certain preparation of snake oil enables the purchaser to lose unwanted fat without change in diet or exercise, and it can be shown in court that this claim is untrue, that is a 'strict liability offence' under the TDA. It is not necessary for the prosecution to show that the advertiser knew the claim was false, so it is possible for a trader to commit this offence without intending to do so. If a misleading description is applied to a medicine, this may have serious consequences, so medicines are specially protected by the Medicines Act 1968.

Medicinal product

The definition of a Medicine is 'Any substance or combination of substances presented for treating or preventing disease in human beings.' Any substance or combination of substances which may be administered to human beings with a view to making a medical diagnosis or to restoring, correcting or modifying physiological functions in human beings is likewise considered a medicinal product. In 1973 reviews of the safety and efficacy of all medicines became mandatory, and only those products that were shown to be safe and effective for specific conditions were licensed by the MHRA, and it was then illegal to make a medicinal claim for a product that did not have a licence. (Regrettably, since 1 September 2006, the rules have been changed. The MHRA may now issue a licence to homeopathic treatments of minor diseases without proper evidence of their efficacy.)

Regulation of claims for CAM treatments

In view of the laws mentioned above, it may seem that it should be easy to control misleading claims for complementary therapies. In practice it is not easy, for several reasons, for which I will give examples below. The law which has, until recently, been most effective is the Medicines Act 1968. It is easy to show if a product has a licence from the MHRA. If it has not, and those promoting it make medicinal claims, then they are breaking the law. If it has a licence then (under the old rules) we could be sure that it had been shown, by proper controlled trials, to be safe and effective for particular conditions.

However, marketing 'alternative' therapies is now big business, and large profits can be made. One of the areas in which the law is open to interpretation concerns 'maintenance of good health' and 'strengthening the immune system'. These might be considered medical claims, but it has been successfully argued in court that such claims are not 'preventing disease' or 'modifying physiological functions', so they do not fall under the requirements of the Medicines Act. I do not know of any prosecutions based on such claims. In practice, such a case would be unlikely to succeed since it is impossible to show, beyond reasonable doubt, that a product did not 'maintain good health' and/or 'strengthen the immune system', since these effects are very difficult to measure accurately. Also, the concept of a 'healthy diet' is widely accepted, and no one advocating a diet rich in fruit and vegetables, and low in sugar, salt and saturated fat, would be expected to show a product licence. But there is a grey area between accepted nutritional advice and commercially promoted snake-oil elixirs. Every high street pharmacy now has shelves packed with food 'supplements' to make your diet even healthier. Usually they do not make overt medicinal claims, but have names such as 'Osteocare' or 'Phytomenopause' or include in the name 'IQ' suggesting the organ or function that would benefit if you take this product.

Pharmacists are bound by the Code of the Royal Pharmaceutical Society. This said that a pharmacist must not 'purchase, sell or supply any medicinal product where the pharmacist has any reason to doubt its safety, quality or efficacy.' This requirement has now been dropped, so the pharmacist is no longer the learned intermediary to help the public to make sound judgements about over-the-counter medication. This is another area in which commercial pressures have triumphed over public interest.

CAM in court for common cures

Magic slimming cures

Misleading claims about weight loss is the commonest type of CAM treatment that has been challenged either by the Advertising Standards Authority (ASA), or in court under the Trades Descriptions Act. This is because very many people would like to become slim quickly, easily, and without tedious dieting or exercising. Products offering this facility are widely advertised, but do not work. Weight loss from week to week is easily measured (unlike 'good health' and a 'strong immune system') so a false claim about weight loss is as easy to prove as that of the publican who gives short measure for drinks.

Below I will review some typical cases that show how the regulatory authorities deal with false claims for products to cause weight loss, and the theories advanced as a basis for these therapies. It is of interest to compare the validity of these theories with those made in support of more up-market CAM treatments.

(1) An electronic exerciser.

An attractive advertisement appeared on page 29 of the *Independent* on 12 October 2005 with the headline 'Get the figure you want for just £19.95!' The text explained 'All over Europe, men and women are choosing the new SlimFly 2005 to tone their body, turn their fat into muscle, and get the figure they want exactly where they want it.' The device is an adhesive patch bearing a battery powered unit that, by 'a wonder of modern electronics' stimulates your underlying muscle 'up to 200 times in 5 minutes.'

I wrote immediately to the ASA to suggest that the advertiser (Bristol Health) should be asked to provide evidence for these claims. They declined to do so, but agreed to withdraw their advertisement. The ASA upheld my complaint, as shown on their website (www.asa.org.uk) on 7 December 2005.

There were two features of this advertisement that were obviously misleading. First, the tiny 'wonder of modern electronics' could not contain a power source that could stimulate underlying muscle. The power source was a single three volt lithium battery, suitable to power a digital watch, but not much more. Second, even if it did stimulate underlying muscle that would not have turned the intervening fat into muscle, as the advertisement implied. Apart from these two flaws the science was quite plausible, and compares favourably with some later examples.

(2) Metabolism booster

Several products claimed to help the slimmer by combining dietary advice with a special ingredient derived from seaweed called fucus. The effect was 'your body's metabolism will activate and actually start to burn off excess calories' creating a 'fat furnace'. It was claimed that 'Autoslim' taken orally would cause 'steady easy weight loss day after day'. Another product—'the amazing anti-fat patch'—administered the fucus transdermally and provided 'simple convenient weight reduction for everyone'. Both products were available by mail order from Jacaranda Ltd in Leicestershire (which later changed its name to Artvert Ltd) and both came with a sheet describing 'Newton's special diet plan'.

A prosecution by Sandwell Trading Standards Office told the magistrates that the active component of fucus was iodine, but the iodine content of the fat patch was below the minimum detectable limit of the Public Analyst, so even if it was all delivered through the skin it would have no significant effect. It was also established that iodine would not activate the metabolism unless the recipient was iodine deficient, which was very improbable in the UK.

The defence was that the diet would cause weight loss if followed, and the product might motivate the customer to follow the diet. The three defendant companies were found guilt of all twelve charges of applying false descriptions to their products, and fined a total of £6000 and ordered to pay £5000 towards the costs of the prosecution.

(3) Starch blockers

A mail-order company which used amazing claims to market food supplements with names such as '*Speedslim*' and '*The Australian*

Anti-fat Miracle' was prosecuted in the Shropshire Crown Court and fined £85,000. Passing sentence, Judge Michael Mander said the false claims about the slimming tablets were a disgraceful and cynical attempt to play on the weakness and vanity of a gullible public.

The *'Australian Anti-fat Miracle'* was said to enable a person within three weeks to lose as much weight as he or she liked without cutting out the foods that person liked, or going on a starvation diet, or taking strenuous exercise. An advertising leaflet explained,

> its unique formula contains a special anti-fat starch blocking ingredient that works by inhibiting enzymes in your digestion thus decreasing your calorific absorption — this blocking action does not cause you unwanted health problems because the valuable vitamins, essential minerals and proteins are still freely absorbed'. Similar claims were made for *'Speedslim'*, which was described as a pure protein legume concentrate. However, studies with ^{13}C-labelled starch showed that, although the ingredient in these products inhibited amylase *in vitro*, it did not work *in vivo* because it was itself digested before it reached the region of the bowel in which starch is digested and absorbed. (Garrow, *et al.*, 1983.)

(4) Fat blockers

Between 1996 and 1998 there were several preparations containing chitosan that were advertised as slimming aids. Chitosan is used by food technologists since it binds fat used in certain confectionaries. It was suggested in the advertisements that, when taken orally, it would bind up to twenty times its own weight of dietary fat in the bowel and thus prevent absorption of this fat. In some products there were also herbal preparations which were claimed to increase the slimming effect by an unspecified mechanism. Birmingham City Council prosecuted Natural Health Supplements Ltd in October 1996 and, after three years of protesting and postponement of trial dates, they pleaded guilty in September 1999. The ASA banned advertisements in the UK that claimed chitosan caused weight reduction, but it is still sold in the USA.

The scientific basis for the use of chitosan is well presented in the report by Pittler *et al.* which showed in a randomised controlled trial that chitosan did not reduce body weight in overweight subjects (Pittler, *et al.*, 1999). It is interesting that this trial was sponsored by Marshtech Ltd, who sold a preparation called 'fat magnet' containing chitosan. This strongly suggests that the vendor sincerely (but wrongly) believed in the efficacy of the product.

CAM: trade, business or profession?

So far all the examples cited above have been about 'alternative' healthcare products or services 'given by a person acting in the course of a trade or business' who has applied a misleading description to what was being sold, so the Trade Descriptions Act applies. What happens if a person applies a misleading description to healthcare products or services he is supplying in the course of a *profession*?

CAM *offered by professionals*

A booklet entitled 'Complementary healthcare: a guide for patients' was issued by the Prince of Wales' Foundation for Integrated Health (FIH) in 2005. This authoritative publication, supported by the Department of Health, lists sixteen 'most widely used' complementary therapies as listed below:

> Chiropractic, Osteopathy, Acupuncture, Herbal medicine, *Aromatherapy, Craniosacral therapy, Healing, Homeopathy, Hypnotherapy, Massage therapy, Naturopathy, Nutritional therapy, Reflexology, Reiki, Shiatsu, Yoga therapy*.

The reader is exhorted to use only 'complementary healthcare provided by a qualified competent practitioner', which implies that such practitioners exist for every therapy, but this is not true. For every therapy shown in italics above there is a paragraph which reads thus:

> Finding an *aromatherapist*
>
> At the moment there is no single body that regulates the *aromatherapy* profession. There are a number of professional associations that practitioners can choose to belong to but an *aromatherapist* is not required by law to belong to a professional association nor to have completed a specified course of training, although many do belong to the organisations listed below.

For other types of CAM therapist substitute *craniosacral therapist* etc. for *aromatherapist*. Otherwise the text is exactly the same.

This is an extraordinary situation. For seventy-five per cent of CAM therapies the practitioners cannot claim professional status since they need not complete a specified course of training, and are not accountable to a single regulating body. To my mind, this means that they are 'acting in the course of a trade or business' and are even less regulated than publicans. In equity, they should be subject to the

Trade Descriptions Act, and required to show that they do not apply misleading descriptions to their goods or services.

Some of these descriptions are highly implausible. I doubt if an average magistrate, presented with a TDA prosecution of a homeopath, could be persuaded that an infinitely diluted solution of something was an effective treatment for a disease similar in effect to that something.

Would he accept that acupuncturists balanced the flow of an unmeasureable energy through certain meridians by inserting needles at exactly the right points, when many studies have shown that any other adjacent point would be just as effective?

Would he believe that pressure on certain reflex points on the hands or feet releases tensions in distant organs and encourages the body's natural healing processes?

Still more bizarre is the claim that very light touch from a craniosacral therapist can rebalance the flow of cerebrospinal fluid within the skull and spinal column. Yet these are all claims made in the FIH guide about unregistered CAM therapies.

I think that if these cases were brought into court the judge would be more likely to echo the comments of Judge Michael Mander and say that these false claims were a disgraceful and cynical attempt to play on the weaknesses and vanity of a gullible public. I do not know, because such cases have never been to court. It seems unjust that the law should punish the vendor of (for example) a 'fat blocker' that he sincerely believed to be effective, when there are CAM practitioners whose claims are far less plausible, but are never tested in front of a judge. In the interest of justice, I would like to see some CAM in court.

References

Garrow, J.S., and others (1983), 'Starch blockers are ineffective in man', *Lancet* 1, 60–1.

Pittler, M.H., and others (1999), 'Randomised double-blind trial of chitosan for body weight reduction', *European Journal of Clinical Nutrition*, 53, 379–81.

Michael Baum and Edzard Ernst

Ethics and Complementary or Alternative Medicine

Introduction

Medical ethics are not absolute codes of conduct that leapt fully formed and immutable from the heads of ancient sages in distant times. Medical ethics in fact demonstrate an uncomfortable plasticity with subtle variations emerging between different ages in history and between different ethnic and cultural groups. The law of the land or medical technology can be important driving forces, but more often than not medical technology runs in advance of our capacity for ethical control and the law is a blunt instrument which may belatedly react to some of the worst medical abuses or as a late reaction to public outcry.

All ethical codes of conduct for the practice of medicine have their bedrock in philosophy and theology. For example, the Hippocratic Oath, which is seldom recited today, probably emerged as a result of the teachings of respect for human rights and dignity at the birthplace of democracy in Athens 400 years before the Common Era. Much of the teaching of Plato and Socrates can be seen reflected in the teachings of Hippocrates. In contrast, contemporary medical ethics is heavily dependent on the teachings of Immanuel Kant of the nineteenth century and his four 'categorical imperatives'—autonomy, beneficence, non-malfeasance and justice.

Contemporary medical problems illustrate the tensions that arise when there is a clash of these categorical imperatives, particularly between distributive justice on one hand and the right to autonomy or self-determination on the other. Furthermore, some of these 'categorical imperatives' clash with ethnic or religious minorities. An example is the current furore regarding the debate between the anti-abortionists (who describe themselves as 'pro-lifers') and those demanding the freedom of the individual to control their families by the use of abortion where necessary (pro-choice).

Thus, even within our narrow Western world of Judeo-Christian belief system, there are many tensions. Yet when we recognise that our society exhibits enormous cultural and religious diversity, the problems are magnified. We can see parallels of this in the debate about CAM. Often we find ourselves talking about systems of faith masquerading as medicine rather than evidence-based practice. This can lead us to the dilemma of allowing, in the name of autonomy, the right to self harm.

Of course, theology plays a much more important role in society than merely underpinning our code of medical ethics. Theology is the basis of faith and faith provides spiritual solace for many of our patients at the time of suffering and comfort when facing the inevitability of death. The practice of religion can contribute to the 'healing' of the spirit, but a clear demarcation has to be made between spiritual healing and healing of the body, although we must leave room to speculate on the links that might exist between a spirit at peace with itself and a body best equipped to heal itself. Nevertheless, from our own experience in medical practice, we must warn that quackery can find fertile soil in filling the gaps vacated by faith in an essentially secular society. The 'new age' belief systems have led to a return to animism, idolatry, witchcraft, astrology and the magic bough. The magic bough (mistletoe) is demonstrating a remarkable reincarnation as Iscador, the most popular 'unproven' remedy for the treatment of advanced cancer.

Ethics is a discipline that asks what is good or bad, right or wrong, moral or amoral. It is of obvious importance, particularly for healthcare. The main ethical principles in medicine are to do more good than harm, to respect patients' autonomy, and to act fairly. Today, no doctor goes through medical training without being taught the essentials of medical ethics. Practitioners of CAM, by contrast, have usually had no or little exposure to such courses. It therefore comes as no surprise that ethical standards in CAM are often found wanting.

The ethical issues in CAM are not fundamentally different from those in conventional medicine. However, the emphasis may be frequently different. Here we will consider the following areas:

- Truth and deception
- Harm and informed consent
- Distributive justice
- Conflicts of interest
- Research ethics

Truth and deception

Truthfulness is an ethical obligation, not just in medicine. Telling the truth to patients can be difficult, particularly when it comes to 'breaking bad news'. In CAM, this scenario rarely occurs. Here 'telling the truth' usually refers to explaining what the current best evidence tells us about the treatments that are being suggested.

But are patients being told the truth? Several studies have tested this by asking CAM practitioners for advice via the internet. The results uniformly indicate that deception is not infrequent in CAM. Recently a British undercover journalist consulted six CAM providers for his (alleged) cancer. Five of the six behaved overtly unethically by deceiving him about the best treatment for his condition. Strikingly similar findings emerged when another UK journalist consulted homeopaths for recommendations about malaria protection.

A related concern involves the use of placebo. Knowingly prescribing placebos to patients would now be considered as paternalistic and an outright deception. Most rational people accept that the most reliable evidence in favour of homeopathy, for instance, can be ascribed to the placebo effect. If clinicians are not aware of that evidence or believe in the absurd and discredited principles of this arcane system despite that evidence then they have failed in keeping up to date with modern medicine. Arguably that in itself might be considered unethical.

Harm and informed consent

Advice which is not supported by good evidence can, of course, seriously harm patients. Our cancer 'patient' (the above-mentioned journalist) would almost certainly have died prematurely had he followed the advice received by the six CAM practitioners he consulted. Even treatments which, by themselves are not harmful, will become life-threatening if they are used as an alternative to effective treatments of serious diseases.

Many people feel attracted to CAM because it is widely portrayed as risk-free, while conventional medicine is regularly associated with serious adverse events. Here we should consider at least two important points. First, not all CAMs are free of risks—just think of the herbal medicines which recently had to be taken off the market because of serious toxicity (e.g. Aristolocia, Kava, Ephedra), or the fact that spinal manipulation has been associated with about 500 published incidences of serious adverse effects, including death. Second, the absolute risk of a treatment is less important than the question whether it generates more good than harm. What really matters is whether a treatment's risks are small compared with the expected benefit. Chemotherapy, for instance, often has significant side-effects. No-one would tolerate such side-effects from a treatment for a common cold. If, however, there is evidence that chemotherapy saves you from dying of cancer, this is a very different matter.

Perhaps the most common ethical dilemma facing the practitioners of CAM, concerns the issue of informed consent. Informed consent is a voluntary, unforced decision, made by a competent or autonomous person, on the basis of adequate information and deliberation, to accept a specific treatment when fully aware of the nature of the treatment, its consequences and risks. There should be no fundamental difference between the information given to a patient in a conventional medical practice compared to that provided in a CAM setting. The problem, of course, is magnified for the 'incompetent' who must now include those who are not gifted with an understanding of the nature of evidence, which probably accounts for most of our patients. If informed consent is to have meaning, then the patient needs to be informed about the uncertainties within which clinicians practise. This applies not only to the clinical trial setting but also to patients treated off protocol in orthodox and alternative medical practice. In medicine we should tolerate only one standard, as double standards would be detrimental, particularly to patients.

In giving permission for a treatment, the patient does not surrender her rights. A failure to fully inform her of the hazards of intended treatments may leave her exposed to liability for criminal charges of negligence or battery.

Yet some 'ethical' practitioners are concerned that full disclosure of all, including rare side-effects of therapy, or the placebo nature of the treatment, may so frighten off a patient from what is judged desirable in their best interests. Therefore they might go against the dictum of beneficence and non-malfeasance. We would argue that this is wrong. As described above, deception by itself denies the patient autonomy by disallowing informed consent.

Distributive justice

What is justice? The shorter Oxford English Dictionary defines justice as 'The quality of being (morally) just or righteous'. Lord Chief Justice Devlin provided a more useful definition: 'We can use the word to mean social justice and then we say that the law is just if it conforms to some social principle, such that all men are equal; that is justice *in rem*.' Note the distinction between the law and justice.

As far as the practice of medicine is concerned Beauchamp makes it clear that our primary concern is distributive justice.

> The principle of justice is really many principles about the distribution of benefits and burdens — to cite one example, an egalitarian theory of justice implies that if there is a departure from equality of distribution of health care benefit and burdens, such a departure must serve the common good and enhance the position of those who are least advantaged in society. (Beauchamp, 1994.)

That definition adheres to the philosophical school of 'utilitarianism' first given voice by Jeremy Bentham. To paraphrase Bentham: the creation of happiness is the main goal in life and all our actions must be for the greatest good for the greatest number. (The danger of this approach, of course, is uncontrolled search for Utopia, which foundered at the Berlin wall.)

It can therefore be predicted that the principle of justice will often be in conflict with the principle of autonomy. In fact, most of the toughest ethical dilemmas we face result from the quite appropriate tension between the ethical principles of justice and autonomy.

As doctors, we have the dual responsibility to care for the individual and to oversee the just distribution of scarce resources in our clinics, our hospital, our health district, our nation and the under-privileged of the third world.

For a start, whenever we are prioritizing our waiting lists we are exercising the principle of justice. We must resist the politician's waiting list initiatives and insist clinical need comes before political expediency. In the inevitable wrangle over hospital resources, always remember that your freedom to carry out as many varicose veins as you damn well like may mean another old lady waits another year for a hip replacement.

Coming back to CAM, let us consider a recent example. Over the period 2003–2006, £20,000,000 was spent refurbishing the Royal London Homeopathic Hospital. The annual revenue costs were about $5,000,000. Yet during this time we had to wait for NICE to adjudicate on the cost effectiveness of two life saving breast cancer drugs (anastrozole and herceptin) followed by a scandalous period of 'post code' prescribing. £20,000,000 alone could have paid for enough of these drugs to save an estimated 600 lives over three years in the UK. The same sums of money might have paid to clear the waiting list for hip replacements, never mind covering the costs of AIDS treatment for children in, say, Malawi if we look beyond our own backdoor in the search for justice. You could go even further and say that the volume of sterile water thrown away in the preparation of homeopathic remedies might have saved the lives of thousands of children dying of dehydration in Somalia over the same period. If the wealthy wish to have the choice of placebo therapy then they can pay for it privately. But if the NHS elects to buy in these 'unproven' remedies then it can only be at the price of ignoring the principle of distributive justice.

Conflicts of interest

By and large, CAM is private medicine; patients in the UK and most other countries pay out of their own pocket directly into the hands of a therapist. As a nation, we spend about £1.6 billion each year on CAM. A single, half-hour treatment might cost £50–100. This creates an obvious conflict. The therapist has a very tangible interest for patients to come back and keep on paying. If your therapist tells you that the treatment is not useful, he would quite simply lose money. If your therapist, on the other hand, persuades you to continue ad infinitum, she is to gain directly and personally. It is hard to think of a more obvious conflict of interest.

This is not a theoretical issue but a very practical concern. Take chiropractors, for instance. They treat acute back pain more often than any other condition. We know that well over ninety per cent of acute back pain will disappear within a matter of 2–3 weeks, regardless of whether we treat it or not. There is little convincing evidence, that chiropractic treatments significantly change any of this. Yet, go to a chiropractor and, in all likelihood, you will receive several x-rays followed by a long series of treatments which are costly (and also often cause side-effects). Eventually your back will be fine again and you may think that is the end of that. But chances are that your therapist has been trained in 'business techniques' which involved pointing out serious misalignments of your spine which would cause long-term damage if not followed up by regular a 'maintenance programme'. This means repeated courses of chiropractic treatments. Yet there is no sound evidence that such an approach does any good at all. CAM therapists are only human and it is hardly surprising that such conflicts of interests cloud their judgements. The loser, unfortunately, is the patient.

Similar conflicts of interest are abundant in CAM. For instance, many investigations have disclosed that customers of health food shops are being advised irresponsibly. At the heart once again is the conflict between the need to make money and the aspiration to improve customers' health. The evidence shows that customers are mislead to buy products which at best will induce a placebo effect and at worse will cause harm. Again, the loser is the patient.

Research ethics

There is a simple rule in medical research: flawed research is unethical. Arguably, much of CAM research is seriously flawed. If a study does not advance our knowledge, if its design is such that the results are unreliable or cannot answer the question posed, if its conclusions do not follow from the data, it is likely to mislead us. In such cases, money and time have been wasted and patients' participation in the study has been abused. When we review the CAM literature we find such flaws all too often. It seems that CAM researchers try to use science to prove their therapy and have little insight in the fact that science is not for proving but for testing. In our opinion, flawed research is likely to be unethical.

As a field, CAM has an ambiguous attitude to rigorous research. Many enthusiasts advocate qualitative over quantitative studies, pragmatic over fastidious trials, or observational over controlled studies. In each case, we have to ask ourselves whether or not this approach is flawed. If the answer is yes, the project could be considered unethical.

Conclusions

There can only be one standard of ethics in health care. Conventional medical practice has a fierce if occasionally dozy watchdog in the General Medical Council (GMC). Why can't we expect the same for

CAM? It is a scandal that so many practitioners of CAM can be involved in the healthcare of our nation without any regulation whatsoever. It is long overdue for the Government to establish an alternative GMC (AGMC) to govern the conduct and ethical integrity of CAM practitioners.

Reference

Beauchamp, T.L. (1994), The 'Four Principles' Approach, in *Principles of Health Care Ethics*, ed. R. Gillon, John Wiley & Sons, Chichester.

Leslie B. Rose and Edzard Ernst

CAM *and Politics*

Practical politics consists in ignoring facts.

Henry Adams (1838–1918)

Of all the UK government's offices of state, perhaps the least desirable is that of Secretary of State for Health. A minister of defence can win wars, a Chancellor of the Exchequer can balance the books, or a minister for education can improve examination results. But a health minister could be excused for feeling like a continual loser. It just is not possible for any state-funded healthcare system to meet everyone's expectations. This is because medical technology advances faster than the availability of funding to deliver the new technology. Patients will always be asking why they can't have the latest drugs and implantable devices. To a minister, health must feel like a big hole into which you throw money, without any prospect of filling it up.

The right to choose

As we write these words, one overriding principle seems to drive public policy on health: patient choice. We will be able to choose which hospital we want for our operations, and are deluged with all sorts of information on performance of those hospitals so that we can make up our minds. We can ask our GP to refer us for a range of therapies, including many of questionable efficacy. A cynic might wonder whether there is an underlying reason for such a policy. Has health become so difficult to manage that some of the responsibility needs to be off-loaded to patients themselves? Of course, it can only be a good thing for patients to take control of their health, instead of ruining it with damaging activities such as smoking and over-eating. But for these two the information for guiding decisions is quite clear. For many others, patients are less well informed by the government, but are still expected to make choices.

Now we should emphasise that, although this essay addresses the political aspects of CAM, it is not party political. Indeed, having been active in this field for many years, the authors cannot find anything to differentiate substantially the main UK political parties on these matters. Rather, we wonder why politicians make the decisions they do, and why they say what they say. There is at least a degree of consistency in the latter. We, the authors, have access to a large amount of correspondence with health ministers, involving both ourselves and others, questioning why this or that form of CAM was promoted or made available on the NHS. The replies from ministers can be summarised largely as 'it's what people want'. Whether it's right for people to be given misleading or incomplete information about what they want seems to be irrelevant. So let's examine in a bit more detail what sort of information politicians are sending out about CAM.

Mixed messages

A good starting point is the Department of Health itself. On its website it still carries information for primary care groups, dated 2000, on CAM.[1] Obviously knowledge has moved on since 2000, but the obsolete information is still there, and no updated version is available. It picks out on page 9 the 'best evidence of effectiveness', for homeopathy in asthma, rhinitis, and hay fever. Let's look at these claims. The best evidence is to be found in meta-analyses and systematic reviews, which summarise the totality of all the clinical trials carried out. For asthma, the current picture is not conclusive (McCarney et al., 2006). A review by homeopaths states that, 'There is not enough evidence to reliably assess the possible role of homeopathy in asthma.' For the other two conditions highlighted in the document, no reviews are available. Yet the Department of Health continues to make the wrong information available, without any warning that it is not current, or any attempt to update it, at the time of writing (August 2007).

In addition to public information from the government itself, various organisations claiming close ties with public health also play a political game. Anyone visiting the website of The NHS Trusts Association might be forgiven for thinking that it is endorsed by or affiliated with the NHS (www.nhsta.org.uk). In reality it is quite separate. This is misleading in itself, but the material it publishes about CAM is even more so. The so-called 'NHS Directory of Com-

[1]   Complementary Medicine: Information for Primary Care Physicians. www.dh.gov.uk/assetRoot/04/01/45/15/04014515.pdf Accessed 6 December 2006.

plementary and Alternative Practitioners' lists a large number of 'therapies' including reiki, reflexology and dowsing. All of these have been subjected to clinical trials—which usually fail to show effectiveness. The Association aligns itself with a website called 'Complementary Alternatives', and shares information with it.[2]

The Association's directory of practitioners is restricted to healthcare professionals on its own site, but freely available to the public on Complementary Alternatives. If you want a crystal therapist or reiki master where you live, you can probably find one there. Unfortunately NHS endorsement is implied by Complementary Alternatives carrying the NHS Trusts Association logo. It surely is very misleading for the directory to be called 'The NHS Directory' when it is nothing to do with the NHS. Curiously, despite being alerted to this abuse, the NHS itself does not seem to care.

The British Broadcasting Corporation enjoys an international reputation for disseminating high quality material. This is justified for most of its output, but commonly not for CAM. News stories frequently lack balance on CAM topics. In early 2006 a story appeared concerning Michael Gearin-Tosh, who had eschewed chemotherapy for cancer in favour of alternative medicine, and had survived. The very high risk of such a decision was not mentioned. A complaint was rejected by the responsible department, so the matter was escalated to the BBC's governors, with supporting testimony from a medical expert. The complaint was again rejected. The BBC also operates a mostly excellent website. However, the CAM section is seriously unbalanced.[3] In the homeopathy area, a laboratory study which had claimed to prove the 'memory of water' (the supposed mechanism by which homeopathy is claimed to work) was cited, without mentioning that it had been discredited and withdrawn by the journal which published it. Many other evidence-free claims are made and, whereas there are lots of links to partisan CAM sites, there are no links to sceptical ones. It took the BBC three months to respond to a complaint which, of course, was rejected. However, the BBC subsequently withdrew the homeopathy page, stating that it was to be updated, and then made several further changes without ever accepting the complaint. These are examples of a public body, funded through taxpayers' money, taking a partisan position on CAM. The argument for independent oversight becomes stronger.

[2]   www.complementaryalternatives.com/default.asp?page
[3]   www.bbc.co.uk/health/healthy_living/complementary_medicine/index.shtml

Selective decision making

In 2000, a Select Committee of The House of Lords published a detailed report on CAM. It recommended more research, particularly into its efficacy and safety, with a substantial investment into dedicated research funds. The government rejected this recommendation and instead opted for funding a series of PhD projects at a fraction of the cost. These projects were then allocated to applicants mostly for sociological projects. Thus virtually no official funding is currently supporting projects which critically evaluate the efficacy and safety of CAM.

While other countries of comparable size and wealth (e.g. Germany) are spending many millions to research CAM, very little CAM research funding is available in the UK. Survey data show that currently the CAM research budget is well below the one per cent margin of the total healthcare research budget of both the NHS and the charitable sector. Considering the many open questions in CAM and the fact that no industry support is available in most areas of CAM, this level of funding is woefully insufficient. The UK's first Chair in CAM suffers badly from this situation. Having attained a reputation for critical assessment (rather than uncritical promotion) of CAM, the unit receives no support from CAM believers nor from the government. It is therefore destined to close in about three years because of lack of funding. Contrast this with the provision by the Department of Health of £20 million for the upgrading of the Royal London Homeopathic Hospital. Indeed the authors have a copy of the business case for this project, and nowhere does it mention evidence-based health outcomes to justify this expense.

But whatever the body of knowledge is on CAM, this needs to be translated into healthcare decisions. The body which does just that is the National Institute for health and Clinical Excellence (NICE). It was set up by the present government to advise on the cost-effectiveness of medicines and other health care technology. Yet over six years after a parliamentary report asked the Government to refer CAMs to NICE, nothing has been done. In a written reply to a question asking why this is the case, the then health minister, Lord Warner, stated that a certain academic unit had been commissioned to select CAM therapies for evaluation, but that no suitable ones had been identified. The said academic unit, on enquiry, denied that any such commission existed. On further written questioning, Lord Warner declined to explain the anomaly. That was all two years ago, at the time of writing, and the last we heard was that NICE is still anxiously awaiting the call to evaluate CAM. It's worth pointing out that, in its response to the parliamentary report in 2000, the government agreed to refer CAM to NICE. How long will ministers take to get around to doing it?

Royal patronage — and related issues

Now we are not conspiracy theorists, but it is interesting to contrast such clear inaction with some rather strange actions by government. In 2005 a CAM lobby group, the Prince of Wales Foundation for Integrated Health, issued its 'Patient Guide to Complementary and Alternative Medicine'. This was in part funded by the Department of Health and the Welsh Office. Readers were surprised that this publication, intended to provide the public with useful information, did not say anything at all about efficacy. The draft guide was sent to one of the present authors (EE), who pointed out in his response that the little information on efficacy (the draft had a table on this subject) was mostly incorrect and offered his team's help in correcting it. After receiving no reply, he wrote a reminder and was finally informed that the Foundation had decided to omit the table (and with it all data on efficacy) altogether.

After the publication of the guide, The Department of Health insisted that information on evidence had never been part of the Foundation's remit. However, the commissioning documents, obtained under the Freedom of Information Act, tell a different story — it clearly was. The Department of Health refused to answer any more questions on the subject, even when the then Health Secretary Dr John Reid was contacted directly.

Not content with rather minor cash support for the Prince of Wales' favourite pastime, the Department of Health quickly shelled out a further £900,000 for the development of schemes to regulate CAM professions in the UK. By now you will not be at all surprised to learn that evidence on efficacy or safety does not feature in the proposed schemes. This closely mirrors the existing legislation by which chiropractic and osteopathy are supposedly regulated — there is no consideration of evidence for either of those.

Despite the UK's ostensibly socialist ruling party, the aristocracy remains very influential. The Prince of Wales is surrounded by a coterie of supporters including various CAM partisans, as well as certain well-known medical and scientific personalities whom one might ordinarily expect to take a more rational view of CAM. The system by which people receive public honours may be arcane to a foreigner, but is transparently clear to anyone observing the Prince's Foundation for Integrated Health. Potential conflicts of interest seem to be tolerated. Michael Fox was for some years simultaneously the chief executive of the Prince's Foundation and a board director of the MHRA (see below). That the Prince has a political agenda is irrefutable. On 23 May 2006 he gave a speech to the World Health Organisation, in which he promoted the use of CAM for serious conditions. He declared:

> I can only urge all health ministers, politicians and Government representatives in this room today to abandon the conventional mindset that sees health as solely the remit of a health department. In ancient China, the doctor was only paid when the patient was well. In modern health systems, perhaps your visible success should depend on health outcomes and the degree to which health has become the responsibility of every single department in your country's Government. Only through collaborative thinking can we paint a complete picture of world healing.[4]

Overseas readers might not realise that, although members of the royal family are specifically barred from taking political action, other aristocrats can legally be active in politics. The House of Lords still has many hereditary peers. The Countess of Mar, whose title was established in the year 1114, speaks regularly in debates in health. She attributes her conviction of CAM's benefits to its ability to cure her of organophosphate poisoning. She relates that, when dipping sheep, some of the dip splashed onto her rubber boot. After that she suffered unspecified 'symptoms', which apparently only a CAM practitioner could resolve. She does not ask why the sheep do not suffer at least as severely – or more so in view of their much greater exposure. This is the kind of unquestioning attitude typical among certain politicians. The cabinet minister Peter Hain MP, formerly Leader of the House of Commons, is a staunch supporter of CAM, and attributes this to the 'cure' of his son's asthma by homeopathy. He does not consider the evidence, which is that homeopathy does not work for asthma. Even a systematic review published by homeopaths shows that to be the case (McCarney *et al.*, 1998). He also admits that his son's diet was changed at the same time, but does not consider that this might have played the major role; and he seems to be ignorant of the well- documented fact that, thankfully, many children simply 'grow out' of being affected by asthma.

---

[4] http://www.princeofwales.gov.uk/speechesandarticles/a_speech_by_hrh_th e_prince_of_wales_on_integrated_healthcare_64.html

Are public servants receiving political pressure?

The regulation of medical products in the UK is the responsibility of the Medicines and Healthcare products Regulatory Agency (MHRA). It is not funded from taxation, but from licence fees. Essentially, a healthcare product is one for which health claims are made, and to be sold it must have a licence issued by the MHRA. To get a licence, a company has to provide information on efficacy, safety and quality, and must pay a fee. Now it's not hard to see that companies choosing to comply with the law are funding the MHRA, while those who choose not to are not. Thus the MHRA has no resources to regulate those who flout the law. A prime example is the proliferation of Chinese medicine shops. These always carry a long list of clear therapeutic claims in the window, such as 'effective treatment for migraine, asthma, arthritis, hypertension ...' If you go into the shop and ask for any evidence in support of these claims, or indeed any information on what the medicines contain, you are unlikely to get anything from the staff. We know, we have tried. While the MHRA has successfully prosecuted several such shops for selling toxic and adulterated material, we are not aware of any attempts to take action against spurious claims. Indeed a formal complaint sent to the MHRA in 2004 about one shop was never addressed. On further enquiry at the time, we were told that the MHRA only had twelve enforcement officers for the whole of the UK, and that ministers were not in favour of taking any stronger action.

Such an example is one of official inertia, but there is another of a deliberate move by the MHRA to accommodate CAM. On 1 September 2006, regulations came into force which permit homeopathic medicines to carry indications on their labels. Hitherto, only such products on the market before 1971, when the 1968 Medicines Act came into force, could carry such claims under a 'licence of right' (in common with all other medicines at the time). All homeopathic products marketed after 1971 are not allowed to carry indications for the diseases they claim to treat. There are currently about 3,000 homeopathic licences, and it is no surprise that the vast majority are licences of right. This contrasts rather sharply with the situation of orthodox medicines, for which virtually no pre-1971 licences exist today. After a public consultation for which a substantial proportion of the responses came from homeopathy companies and interest groups, the proposals were laid before parliament four days before the summer recess, and came into force over five weeks before MPs returned to Westminster. There was thus no opportunity for debate.

Interestingly, the MHRA said that there were no strong public health reasons for taking any action, and that the only reason for not revoking all homeopathic licences was the expectation of pressure from the homeopathy companies. The MHRA clearly documented its desire to expand the homeopathy industry, and instead of requiring companies to provide clinical trial based efficacy data (which the MHRA admitted was not possible), 'non-scientific data' based on the homeopathic tradition could be accepted. Naturally there was a huge reaction to all this, with many learned societies and leading scientists strongly criticising the MHRA, whose mission statement includes the words 'ensuring that medicines and medical devices work'. Apparently this now need not involve science. The MHRA has taken very similar action over a herbal remedy, arnica gel. New labelling allows this product to be promoted for bruising and other minor trauma. At the time, only one controlled clinical trial had been carried out on this product, showing no evidence of efficacy. A distinguished colleague of ours, a professor of pharmacology, has repeatedly asked the MHRA to address the contention that the labelling is misleading to consumers, to no avail.[5] No amount of direct questioning can extract anything other than evasive responses. Meanwhile in a news release the MHRA commended the manufacturer of arnica gel for obtaining a product licence under the new rules. It is worth pointing out that the chief executive of the MHRA, Professor Kent Woods, and its chairman Professor Sir Alasdair Breckenridge, are both members of the British Pharmacological Society, which has issued a statement condemning the homeopathy regulations.

Playing the political game

We have already referred to letters from the health minister Lord Warner, with regard to his failure to refer CAMs to NICE for cost-effectiveness appraisal. That correspondence established a pattern which ministers seem to follow habitually. When asked a difficult question, they usually respond by seemingly misunderstanding, and answering a question which has not been asked. When pressed for an answer, they again divert the flak by referring, usually at great length, to actions they have taken which bear only tenuous relevance to the question. We are continually amazed at the ability of politicians to write many words without saying anything.

---

[5]   www.ucl.ac.uk/Pharmacology/dc-bits/quack.html#mhra36

The final stage is usually one of exasperation, when the politician refuses to continue the exchange on the basis that it has gone on for long enough.

To illustrate stage one of the process, we were recently sent a copy of a letter from the health minister Caroline Flint, addressed to a member of the public who had challenged the government's funding of homeopathy. The minister responded by referring the correspondent to the Faculty of Homeopathy. Could any intelligent person have so misunderstood the question? Lord Warner, as set out above, is a past master at stages two and three. Stage three is also epitomised by the exchanges over the 'Patient Guide' to CAM, which culminated with Dr Reid declining to reply to questions, and delegating them to civil servants, who eventually stopped responding.

In similar vein, the new Health Minister Lord Hunt recently replied thus to a question about fraudulent 'psychic surgeons':

> There are currently no plans to extend statutory regulation to other professions, such as psychic surgery. We expect these professions to develop their own unified systems of voluntary self-regulation. If they then wish to pursue statutory regulation, they will need to demonstrate that there are risks to patients and the public that voluntary regulation cannot address.

Now the question had included the example of one Stephen Turoff, who had already been exposed on national television, faking invasive procedures by palming bits of wet cotton wool and other theatrical props. Yet the minister ignored the matter of fraudsters exploiting very sick and vulnerable people, and was not in the least interested in the matter of evidence to support outrageous claims. The last sentence is astonishingly disingenuous. Does Lord Hunt really expect people faking surgical treatment to come to him and say 'Well, we are sorry but there are risks, so we would like to be regulated please'? It's hard to believe that even politicians can be this stupid.

But perhaps quite a lot are. In May 2007 several NHS primary care trusts announced major reductions in referrals of patients to the five NHS homeopathic hospitals. Most of them cited the need for evidence -based clinical decisions. This of course stimulated a major protest from the hospitals themselves and their supporters. Part of this was the tabling of a motion in the House of Commons, supporting the hospitals and recognising their 'positive contribution made to the health of the nation'. It listed many conditions for which there is no evidence of benefit from homeopathy. Amazingly, this attracted support from 197 MPs, almost one third of the whole House. One signatory was the former chair of the House's Science and Technology Committee, and a former scientist of note. It seems that politics can have a very pernicious effect on critical thinking.

But does it matter?

In an interview given to the magazine *New Scientist*, and published on 4 November 2006, Prime Minister Tony Blair said: 'My advice for the scientific community would be, fight the battles you need to fight. I wouldn't bother fighting a great battle over, say, homeopathy. It's not going to determine the future of the world.' This typifies a quite widely held view that irrational beliefs are not important, and put into the context of the whole interview, shows how poorly understood science is by many politicians. Blair sees science as a tool for building economic competitiveness, not as a system for uncovering knowledge.

We must revisit the opening themes of this piece. We are in receipt of many letters from government ministers which continue to place patient choice above telling the truth about medical treatments. Direct challenges to misleading government information and policies are usually ignored. Politics has become market led, with politicians following public opinion, instead of leading with robust and creative policies, communicated with integrity. By misrepresenting such evidence as does exist, and by failing to support proper research, the government is submerging the true benefits which some CAMs may have in a flood of pseudoscience (Ernst *et al.*, 2006).

Panel 1: Tips and tools for dealing with politicians and public servants

In the UK, the prevailing protocol is that a member of the public is expected to question government ministers via letters to their Member of Parliament. Thus the vigour with which a question is pursued is highly dependent on how important the MP thinks it is. But this is not an absolute rule and, for example, an MP without an interest in a subject may refer the constituent to another MP. This can be useful, as there are not many MPs who know much about evidence-based medicine (EBM). Indeed, there is an all-party CAM group, comprising mostly uncritical supporters, but no group supporting EBM. Also, of course, any member of the public can write directly to a minister. Generally though, the reply will come from a civil servant. If you want a letter signed by the minister, you will have to go via your MP.

Dealing with public servants can be monumentally frustrating, as we have noted elsewhere in this essay. But you can at least talk directly to them. Websites such as those of the MHRA and Department of Health publish contact details for people with key responsibilities. It is worth telephoning, as you can get a much better idea of what people are thinking. For example, in conversation with one MHRA official, some key admissions were made about the regulation of homeopathy, but permission to quote these was refused. This made it clear that political pressure was being brought to bear on public servants.

Panel 2: Obtaining public information

We have mentioned here the Freedom of Information Act 2000, under which some of the documents we discuss were obtained. Since the Act came into force in 2005, public bodies have become increasingly reluctant to release information. We do not propose to provide a guide to utilising the Act here, as detailed information is available on the websites of the Campaign for Freedom of Information (www.cfoi.org.uk) and the Office of the Information Commissioner (www.ico.gov.uk). Briefly, it has become common for public bodies to claim a number of exemptions allowed under the Act, typically concerning commercial sensitivity, and communications with the royal household. The key point here is that most exemptions are subject to a public interest test. This means that, if on balance the public interest is served by releasing information, it must be released. If the public body will not comply with the Act, you have the right to request an internal review, and after that to complain to the Information Commissioner. All this can, of course, take months, and public bodies are becoming adept at using delaying tactics, while the government is seeking to impose further constraints on the release of information.

References

Ernst, E., Pittler, M.H., Wider, B., Boddy, K. (2006), *The Desktop Guide to Complementary and Alternative Medicine* (Edinburgh: Mosby/Elsevier).

McCarney, R.W., Linde, K., Lasserson, T.J. (1998), 'Homeopathy for chronic asthma', *Cochrane Database of Systematic Reviews 1998*, Issue 1. http://www.cochrane.org/reviews/en/ab000353.html

Edzard Ernst

Integrated Medicine?

It used to be called alternative, then complementary medicine or complementary/alternative medicine (CAM); now the term integrated (or integrative in the US) medicine is the new buzz word. But integrated medicine is not identical with CAM. The word implies a marriage of alternative and conventional approaches; some speak of 'the best of both worlds' and point out that it is unique—a chance to improve healthcare which we never had before.

In this essay, I will first demonstrate that a historical precedent does exist and subsequently submit the concept of integrated medicine to a critical analysis. Finally, I will discuss what integrated medicine can mean in practice.

A historical precedent

Beginning in the mid-nineteenth century, a general nature-orientated movement had gripped most of Europe. It led to a division between scientific and 'natural medicine', i.e. CAM. The 'natural medicine movement' was driven predominantly by lay people. In Germany they were organized in associations, which, by the 1930s had about half a million members and 5–10 million non-registered supporters. Conventional medicine was deemed to be in a deep crisis, and 'natural medicine' was seen by many as the solution. In 1933, the number of lay-therapists had grown to be roughly equal to that of physicians registered in Germany, a situation similar to the present one in the UK.

The healthcare profession of 'Heilpraktiker' (literal translation: healing practitioner) was created to unify all the non-medical practitioners under Nazi rule. The Nazis believed that unifying all of German medicine into the 'Neue Deutsche Heilkunde' (literal translation: new German healing practice) would help to overcome the schism in medicine and lead healthcare out of the crisis. Their strategy was to legalise and appease the lay-practitioners by giving them the new and official status of 'Heilpraktiker'. In parallel, the medical profession was to be extensively trained in natural medicine. Dr G. Wagner, the Reich's chief medical officer, wrote in 1935: 'If today we want to construct a new German healing practice, then its basis cannot be that formed by the exact sciences but its basis must be our national socialist world view'. The 'Neue Deutsche Heilkunde' was designed to integrate science and CAM.

In 1939, the profession of the 'Heilpraktiker' became officially instituted and included all lay practitioners of the time. They were given similar rights and standing as physicians (thus they were happy). However, they were not licenced to educate a next generation of 'Heilpraktiker'. Therefore they would become extinct within only a few decades (thus the doctors were happy). Goebbels called the 'Heilpraktiker' law the 'cradle and the grave' of a new profession. The reason why 'Heilpraktiker' still exist today is that, after the war, the 'Heilpraktiker' profession challenged and overturned the prohibition to educate future practitioners.

A show-case example of the new medicine was a hospital in Dresden, named after Rudolf Hess (Hitler's deputy). Hess, like several other 'Nazi VIPs', was an outspoken proponent of homeopathy. The concept of the hospital was the integration of mainstream medicine and CAM. It was meant to be a model for German medicine of the future. Hess demanded of the German medical professions 'to test in an unbiased way treatments that had so far been rejected'. This quote is revealing: good evidence that CAM did more good than harm did evidently not exist.

As it turned out, the course of history and the absence of good evidence limited the impact of this experiment. After his death, the Reich's chief medical officer, Dr G. Wagner, an ardent supporter of the 'Neue Deutsche Heilkunde' was replaced by Dr Conti who showed much less interest. Hess was declared a traitor and, in 1941, the hospital was re-named 'Gerhard-Wagner Krankenhaus'. The Second World War forced German medicine to concentrate on the essentials, i.e. treatments with well-documented efficacy—and that excluded CAM.

Despite the obvious political differences, the parallels of the 'Neue Deutsche Heilkunde' and today's integrated medicine are obvious.

- Both movements were initially driven by the lay public.
- The proportion of lay healers to doctors is similar.

- In both instances there was much talk of a crisis in (orthodox) medicine.

- Integration did not evolve naturally but was politically enforced.

- In both instances there was not enough evidence to justify integration.

A critical analysis of integrated medicine

Similar to 'Neue Deutsche Heilkunde', the current term integrated medicine is ambiguous and has two distinctly different meanings. Integrated medicine 'views patients as whole people with minds and spirits as well as bodies and includes these dimensions into diagnosis and treatment'. Such definitions demonstrate that integrated medicine is essentially medicine which follows the ethical imperative to maintain human relations in healthcare (see also M. Baum's essay in this volume). It simply highjacks the concept of holistic healthcare.

The creation of the term 'integrated medicine' also implies that conventional physicians are incapable of a whole person approach. It thus perpetuates the myth that conventional healthcare professionals see their patients as malfunctioning elbows, blocked arteries etc, and gives the impression that scientific medicine and holism are incompatible. In truth, they complement each other in perfect harmony. Throughout history physicians have excelled in combining both (see also M. Fitzpatrick's essay in this volume). Virtually all definitions of medicine, new or old, emphasize its holistic nature. If we want a more holistic approach to our current healthcare systems, we should work directly towards this aim rather than confusing people through the creation of new terminology. Integrated medicine, by its first definition, is merely the duplication of concepts which have always been at the heart of medicine. The concepts are essential; the new term, however, is superfluous and arguably counter-productive.

The second, more widely appreciated definition of integrated medicine means

> the use of different therapies, including both complementary medicine and conventional medicine and different healthcare agencies and practitioners, in a co-coordinated and mutually supportive programme of care for the greatest benefit of the individual patients.

Rees and Weil have formulated it a little differently: 'practicing medicine in a way that selectively incorporates elements of CAM into comprehensive treatment plans.' And the Prince of Wales repeatedly spoke of 'the best of both worlds'.

The driving forces behind this second concept are rarely explicit. Implicitly they are based on data demonstrating that large and growing numbers of patients try CAM, and that CAM-users come from the more privileged sections of the population. This, proponents argue, is an injustice; to re-establish justice, we need an equal distribution of power between the 'politically dominant' (i.e. conventional medicine) orthodoxy and the suppressed heterodoxy (i.e. CAM). Essentially this argument uses popularity as a justification for integration. A document from the Prince of Wales' Foundation states that, 'given patients' demands and utilization of CAM therapies, despite the lack of evidence, there is an increasing need to address how CAM therapies can be integrated into conventional medical systems'.

What about this 'lack of evidence'? Proponents of integrated medicine seem to want to simply ignore this question. But can we? Some CAM modalities are supported by reasonably good evidence, most have not yet been adequately investigated to allow firm conclusions, others clearly do not generate more good than harm and some seem too implausible to even justify the expenditure of scientific testing. Integrating CAM where it is evidence-based is logical, ethical and necessary. But if we start integrating therapies (complementary or conventional) with an uncertain risk-benefit balance, our healthcare systems might become more equitable at the expense of getting less effective and more costly. Standards would not rise but would inevitably fall. The integration of nonsense must result in nonsense.

CAM enthusiasts believe that users of CAM feel satisfied with it and insist that 'we must give patients choice ...' (see also Hazel Thornton's essay in this volume). But survey data are clearly no substitute for the results of carefully controlled clinical trials, and patient satisfaction suggested by (often low quality) surveys is not the same as evidence of a positive risk-benefit balance. In the words of Gordon Brown:

> it is wrong to regard patients as consumers. They lack relevant information. They may not even know they are ill, be poorly informed of available treatments, be reliant on others to understand the diagnosis, and be uncertain about the effectiveness of different medical interventions—all of which places them in a less influential position than consumers of retail goods.

Others might counter that the primacy of patient choice is unquestionable. The contradiction is, however, only an apparent one. Patient choice does not mean that healthcare professionals (or anyone else) should encourage the use of untested or disproven treatments. Healthcare professionals have an obligation to direct their patients towards therapies that have been adequately tested and demonstrably generate more good than harm; we must be sure that new treatments are worth while before they are integrated into routine care. Of course, clinicians are merely advisers of patients — but responsible advice must be based on sound evidence. If integrated medicine is understood in this way it becomes synonymous with evidence-based medicine. Again the term is disclosed as superfluous and counter-productive.

Integrated medicine in action

'The best of both worlds' is the beautiful theory which can easily be slain by ugly facts. In the final section of this essay, I will briefly ask what integrative medicine means in practice. When addressing this question, one is struck by the lack of systematic research on this issue. In fact, it is hard to find any systematic evidence at all. Here are a few anecdotal examples of what integrated medicine means in everyday practice.

The current chairman (Dr Michael Dixon) of the UK NHS Alliance, an umbrella body for general practitioners, is a vocal proponent of integrated medicine. On the occasion of an initiative to recruit general practitioners to the concept, he was reported to have stated the following: 'We want GPs to realise if a patient has a frozen shoulder you can go down the traditional route and give them a tablet, give them physiotherapy, or send them to a surgeon. Alternatively, devil's claw and acupuncture are also proven to work' (*Sunday Times*, 14 August 2005). I know of no good evidence that either of these CAM modalities are effective treatments for a frozen shoulder. But few proponents of integrated medicine seem to be all that concerned about double standards. In fact, that is exactly what Dr Dixon (on a different occasion in 2003) advocated: 'We are going to have to invent our own set of rules and not accept anything as a given' (Dixon, 2003).

The preamble of the US *Journal of Complementary and Integrative Medicine* gives another interesting clue as to what integrated medicine actually does mean: 'This approach includes … the use of herbal medicines … in improving the efficacy and/or reducing the toxicity profile of drugs.' Again I would question the evidence-base for this statement. In fact, the existing evidence shows the opposite: many herbal medicines interact with prescription drug to the detriment of the patient.

Israel Barken MD runs a web site entitled 'What is integrative medicine and how can prostate cancer patients benefit from it?' There he states that 'lycopenes are excellent for prostate cancer patients'.[1] These chemicals found in tomatoes and other plants may have a role in cancer prevention but I am not aware that they are useful for treating cancer.

Dr Joseph Pizzorno is a US proponent of integrated medicine. In an interview with 'News Target. Com', he advocated glucosamine sulfate, vitamin C and lipoic acid for pain and stiffness after playing football.[2] Yet there is no sound evidence that this would help.

The 'Integrated Medicine Wheel' runs a website where it is stated that antibiotics which have lost their power through bacterial resistance become effective again when combined with 'certain herbs'.[3] I know of no such evidence and fear that such advice might seriously endanger the health of patients.

Under the heading 'Congress on Integrative Medicine kicks off in Beijing', we find another revealing example on the World Wide Web: 'integrative medicine to cure white blood corpuscle deficiency, hepatitis, cardiovascular disease, burns and fractures'.[4] On 'Barnes and Noble.com' the following statement can be found: 'back and neck pain benefit from homeopathy'. Do I need to repeat it? There is no evidence for such claims.

The message that emerges from these selected examples (one could find many more) seems clear: integrated medicine is by no means 'the best of both worlds'. Often it means the substitution of demonstrably effective treatments by remedies which are unproven or even disproven. Integrated medicine promotes CAM no matter what the evidence says. This is a cynical violation of the principles of evidence based medicine at the expense of effective and cost-effective healthcare. The looser in all this, I fear, would be the patient.

---

[1]   www.prostatepointers.org/barken/barken2.html
[2]   www.newstarget.com/007134.htm (accessed 21/01/08)
[3]   www.collinge.org/imw.htm (accessed 21/01/08)
[4]   www.barnesandnoble.com (accessed 21/01/08)

Conclusion

History repeats itself. The present boom in integrated medicine has many similarities with the concept of the 'Neue Deutsche Heilkunde' seventy years ago. That concept failed, not least because there was no good evidence to support it. If today's integrated medicine movement continues to ignore the importance of a sound evidence -base, it will also fail. Meanwhile the uncritical integration of unproven or disproven treatments into routine healthcare is a significant disservice to patients who have a right to be treated with the most effective treatments available at any given time.

References

Brown, G. (2003), Quoted in Dean, M.: UK Health Secretary promises more choice for NHS patients, *Lancet*, 362: 458.

Dixon, M. (2003), CAM in the context of primary care. Presentation to Developing clinical governance for CAM in primary care, a Kings Fund Seminar, London, 30 January 2003.

Ernst, E., Pittler, M.H., Wider, B., Boddy, K. (2006), *The Desktop Guide to Complementary and Alternative Medicine* (2nd edn) (Edinburgh: Elsevier Mosby).

HRH Prince Charles (2001), 'The best of both worlds', in *British Medical Journal*, 322, 181.

Rees, L. and Weil, A. (2001), Integrated medicine. *British Medical Journal*, 162: 133–40.

G.V.R. Born

Homeopathy in Context

In 2005 a *Lancet* article compared placebo controlled clinical trials of homeopathy and conventional medicine (Shang *et al.*, 2005), and concluded that any effects of homeopathy were merely placebo. This elicited an authoritative assertion from the homeopathic community that controlled clinical trials are inapplicable as a tool for testing homeopathic efficacy (the *Guardian*, 29 August 2005). The scientific medicine community is bound to come to the same conclusion but for an entirely different reason, namely that the basis for the therapeutic claims of homeopathy is incompatible with the scientific basis of undoubtedly effective drugs. That both sides reach the same conclusion should put an end once and for all to the submission of homeopathic preparations to controlled clinical trials: they cannot be *expected* to show anything more than placebo effects.

Because homeopathy claims to make sick people better by administering medicines it is of all the so-called alternative medicines closest to the science of pharmacology. Pharmacology is rigorously based on its neighbouring sciences of chemistry, physiology, pathology, immunology and so on, and admirably successful in producing drugs that actually do make people better. Basic to effective drug therapy are dose-response relationships compatible with the laws of science (see e.g. Kenakin, 1997). Like all sciences, pharmacology is subject to verifiability and falsifiability and progresses continually.

In contrast, homeopathy is based on unchanging dogma which excludes any possibility of progress. The dogma, ever since its invention by Samuel Hahnemann around 1810, states that *similia similibus curantur*—like cures like—that is to say a disease is to be treated by administering minute doses of a substance which produces symptoms in the healthy person similar to those produced by the disease itself. Furthermore, the homeopathic principle of *potencies* states that preparations retain curative activity even after they are serially diluted to such an extent that essentially none of the supposed remedy remains (see Clark, 1940). As nothing ever changes in homeopathy, it has been pointed out that Hahnemann (1755–1843) would be able to pass all homeopathy examinations today without difficulty, whereas the greatest medical figures of his century such as Joseph Lister (1827–1912), Rudolf Virchow (1821–1902), Robert Koch (1843–1910), could not possibly pass today's medical finals. Hahnemann can be excused from promulgating his mistaken ideas at a time when the biomedical sciences were in their infancy. No such excuse is available to his present-day disciples, whose adherence to the original dogma shows a mindset impervious to scientific facts as well established as those providing us with electric light.

The irreconcilable differences between homeopathy and scientific therapeutics are illustrated by representative publications from both sides. Books such as *Classical Homeopathy* by Margery Blackie published in 1986 continue to be used by homeopathic practitioners as a basis for treatments. There is no way in which effects of the preparations described in this publication could be scientifically demonstrable. By contrast, the scientific bases of anaesthetics, analgesics, antibiotics, anti-hypertensives, lipid-lowering agents, hormone therapies and so much else are documented in established textbooks such as *The Pharmacological Basis of Therapeutics* by L.S. Goodman and A.G. Gilman. First published in 1941 and now in its eleventh edition (2005), this book is totally updated every few years as new knowledge accumulates. A recent Supplement to the *British Journal of Pharmacology* (North, 2006) reviews outstanding British contributions to these therapeutic achievements. With all this in mind, the unchanging doctrines of homeopathy might be considered an affront to the immense efforts of hundreds of scientists devoted to the elucidation of the complex cellular and molecular systems on which real drugs depend.

Nowadays, homeopathy should be no more than a quaint, essentially harmless, historical footnote. However, it could well become a serious matter through practitioners failing to recognize potentially dangerous diseases, which would thereby be brought to medical attention too late for effective treatment. Nowadays, the promotion of homeopathy as more than a kind of placebo is indefensible; and for Universities to offer the scientific degree of BSc in Homeopathy is disgraceful (Colquhoun, 2007).

A senior homeopathy practitioner (the *Guardian* 29 August 2005) has claimed that the popularity of homeopathy is increasing. This would be just another example of the worrying growth of irrationalities, and would be detrimental not only for individuals but also for the NHS in so far as it has been providing money for homeopathic practices from the public purse. The trouble is that most people know too little science to recognize the nonsense that is homeopathy. For the same reason, people fail to understand why scientific medicine has still no cures for common rheumatic and nervous diseases nor indeed for most cancers. All medical achievements are inevitably limited by the relevant knowledge at any given time. Lack of awareness of these limits subjects scientific medicine to excessive expectations, which is paradoxical because the reason for excessive expectations is precisely the established successes of *scientific* medicine. It is when expectations are not fulfilled that alternative medicines beckon; and this is undoubtedly the main reason why homeopathy persists.

Unfortunately there are also two other reasons: doctors in the NHS are almost always pressed for time, whereas homeopaths make a point of giving adequate time to those who seek them out. Furthermore, not everyone may wish to know how their body works, because this knowledge could make one afraid of all the things that might go wrong. Whatever the reason, the appeal of baseless practices such as homeopathy becomes understandable: we all look for help in the face of pain, disease and death. But we all, including homeopathic practitioners, should be profoundly grateful for living in the era in which unquestionably effective treatments based on scientific knowledge are enabling ever increasing numbers of us to enjoy healthier and longer lives.

What can be done to counteract the persistence of homeopathy? Its unwarranted claims must be continuously exposed. The diversion of public money from the proper purposes of the NHS must be stopped. Homeopathic practioners with proven abilities to enhance patients' sense of well-being (see *Magic or Medicine* by Buckman and Sabbagh, 1993) might be designated 'placebo therapists'. And finally, 'education, education, education' must ensure that everyone from childhood on acquires sufficient biological knowledge to help him or her distinguish between valid and invalid therapies. Experience tells us that such a learning process is both appealing and fulfilling all the way through education.

References

Blackie, M. (1986), *Classical Homeopathy*, ed. C. Elliot and F. Johnson (London: Beaconsfield).

Buckman, R. and Sabbagh, K. (1993), *Magic or Medicine?* (London: Macmillan).

Clark, A.J. (1940), *Applied Pharmacology* , 7th edn (London: Churchill), p. 3.

Colquhoun, D. (2007), 'Science degrees without the science', *Nature*, London,446, 373–4.

Goodman, L.S. and Gilman, A.G. (2001), *The Pharmacological Basis of Therapeutics* (10th edn), (New York: McGraw-Hill).

Kenakin, T. (1997), *Pharmacologic Analysis of Drug-Receptor Interaction*, 3rd edn (New York: Lippincott-Raven).

North and Rang (2006), *British Journal of Pharmacology 75th Anniversary Supplement*, ed. R.A. North and H.P. Rang.

Shang, A., Huwiler-Müntener, K., Nartey, L., Jüni, P., Dörig, S., Sterne, J.A., Cpewsner, D., Egger, M. (2005), 'Are the clinical effects of homoeopathy placebo effects? Comparative study of placebo-controlled trials of homoeopathy and allopathy', *Lancet*, 366, 726–32.

Terry Polevoy

Chiropractic

Science, religion or political movement?

Historical precedence

Chiropractic began in the last two decades of the nineteenth century in Davenport, Iowa by a transplanted Canadian grocer named Daniel David Palmer. He was a supporter of religious revivalism, yet he also believed in animal magnetism and spiritualism in what was then the Bible Belt of the US Midwest. The sign on his door read 'D.D. Palmer Cures Without Medicine'. He thrived by advertising widely, and used huge billboards to promote his clinic that at one time had 40 exam rooms.

After he claimed to cure a janitor of his deafness by banging on his spine, he came to believe that he had found the cure for 95% of all illnesses. He called the misalignments of the spine 'subluxations', and that term has continued to be the very foundation of almost all of chiropractic for over 110 years.

His prowess was in making a lot of money by seeing 100 patients in a short afternoon in his clinic. In the early twentieth century the concept of Innate Intelligence was added to the chiropractic belief system. He claimed that only chiropractors could keep the nerves in tune. His theories changed many times over the years, but they were never based on scientific facts. It was D.D. Palmer who introduced the concept of treating infants because their spine was subluxed during the birthing process.

Today, many of the original theories, that some would call religious beliefs, have not been dropped. Many chiropractic schools still teach the 'philosophy' of chiropractic and refuse to recognize the absurd claims made by this huckster. Unfortunately, what began as a wacky back-cracking idea to cure the world of all of its illnesses has grown around the world. How and why this happened is a mystery.

Data is not the plural of anecdote:

As famed scientist Robert Park said so eloquently,

> If modern science has learned anything in the past century, it is to distrust anecdotal evidence. Because anecdotes have a very strong emotional impact, they serve to keep superstitious beliefs alive in an age of science. The most important discovery of modern medicine is not vaccines or antibiotics, it is the randomized double-blind test, by means of which we know what works and what doesn't. Contrary to the saying, 'data' is not the plural of anecdote. (Park, 2003)

Chiropractic for tens of thousands of practitioners around the world is nothing more than a way to provide what they believe is the right choice for their patients. Whether or not what they learned in chiropractic colleges has sustained the test of time really means little to them. In the US chiropractors pay tens of thousands of dollars to attend schools that in some instances have been not proved to be exactly what they expected. To avoid governmental regulatory oversight over their advertising and avoid payment of taxes, these programs are universally established as non-profit organizations. There have been a number of lawsuits against these schools in recent years, and the largest one, Life University in Marietta, Georgia, had its accreditation revoked for failure to teach differential diagnosis and promoting a subluxation based insurance fraud scheme. As a whole, chiropractic students have the highest default rate for loans in North America.[1]

Chiropractors have been overproduced by all chiropractic schools, including those with questionable credentials. It matters little to most chiropractic regulating bodies that their brethren continue to flood the market. The people who are the most excited by the thousands of students are of course the chiropractic vendors of machines, furniture, books, and other paraphernalia. Mainstream medical publishers now kowtow to the pseudo-scientific poppycock that is still rampant in chiropractic.

Despite the fact that just a few universities around the world have associated themselves with chiropractic education to try to bring it into the twenty-first century, the inferior training received by most chiropractic students continues to be the accepted 'standard', at least in the US. Canada still only had two chiropractic colleges, one in Ontario and one in Quebec. A few years ago, York University, Canada's third largest school, soundly rejected an opportunity to swallow up the Canadian Memorial Chiropractic College.

---

[1] References for this paragraph: http://chirobase.org/03Edu/webclaims.html http://www.prweb.com/releases/2006/5/prweb383327.htm

Benefits vs. Risks

Exactly what are the claimed benefits of chiropractic? It all depends on what you consider chiropractic to begin with. If you restrict their practices to disorders of the spine and musculoskeletal system there may be small benefits to some treatments of low back pain. Fortunately, most acute low back pain gets better within a few weeks, with or without any treatment at all. Studies reviewed by *NCCAM (National Center for Complementary and Alternative Medicine)* has the following to say about spinal manipulation for low back pain:

> The studies all found at least some benefit to the participants from chiropractic treatment. However, in six of the eight studies, chiropractic and conventional treatments were found to be similar in effectiveness. One trial found greater improvement in the chiropractic group than in groups receiving either sham manipulation or back school. Another trial found treatment at a chiropractic clinic to be more effective than outpatient hospital treatment.

The present state of chiropractic promotion

The main problems with chiropractic today are not just that their profession has relied on D.D. Palmer's original work. Over the last hundred years or so, thousands of chiropractic self-promoters have created their own versions of what they say works. Pick up any chiropractic magazine that most chiropractors leave in their waiting rooms and you get the idea that the philosophy (or pseudo-religion) of their profession is still quite prominent. Just check your local newspaper and you will see their ads that promote their free information seminars to drag patients into their offices. Go to a shopping mall, or health fair and you will often see groups of chiropractors with their 'free office visit' coupons after they do a public back screening.

Some of the worst examples of chiropractic promotions are the radio shows, often masked as news, that permeate the airwaves. I've collected hundreds of hours of these shows, including some TV spots from around the world, and it is amazing what they say and what they promise they can do. Complaints to the media moguls just fall on deaf ears because they are hungry for advertising revenue.

Some of the most powerful chiropractic promoters over the years have been Scientologists. They hire people who they hand-pick, and then force them to proselytize not just for chiropractic, but for Scientology, too. It's really not that hard to pick them out, they don't hide behind a dark curtain of anonymity. Just try putting in Scientology and chiropractic into any search engine. As a personal note, one of my employees once worked for a chiropractic Scientologist and she quit when advised that as a condition of her employment, she would have to toe the party line.

Why do they have to promote?

One of the adages for any business success is that they locate where the patients are. It's the old 'location, location, location' slogan that drives the 'business' of chiropractic. But there is a problem with this concept. If there is a chiropractor in every strip mall, and professional building and real estate agents and banks who are willing to work with a young professional to get them started, many of them will be forced into bankruptcy or default on their student loans within a few months or years.

Instead of a thriving practice, with patients stacked up in the waiting room like cattle, many operators are staring at an empty office. What was once a niche practice area is now nothing more than an expensive, and in my opinion, an unnecessary commodity. While insurance coverage is mandated in many areas, so that everyone could be covered, it does not guarantee that their appointment books will be filled with eager patients. Don't forget that not everyone who seeks relief for their strained back goes to a chiropractor. About 10 years ago, there were 50,000 chiropractors in the US. In the next six years the projections for the number of practicing chiropractors will be up to 70,000. They will have to compete with 185,000 physiotherapists, 117,000 massage therapists, and 27,000 acupuncturists.

It's a living?

In order to earn a living, chiropractors and their professional promoters have added a large number of other modalities to support their practices. These include homeopathy, acupuncture, live cell microscopy, nutrition, herbology, and the promotion of a host of unproved devices that are used to recruit and keep patients.

Many companies are marketing irrationally formulated supplement products exclusively or primarily through chiropractors. Most chiropractors who recommend supplements sell them to their patients at two to three times their wholesale cost.

Some chiropractic techniques and devices are even promoted to pregnant mothers and in the newborn nursery. Techniques may even include rectal or vaginal examinations that have resulted in a significant number of chiropractors who have been charged with sexual assault.

Some of the most mysterious practices now embraced by a growing number of chiropractors don't even involve the manipulation of the spine. For instance, claims are made by some practitioners of *Network Spinal Analysis* that all they have to do is to wave their hands over the body or gently touch the spine or neck and they can assist the body to heal itself.

One bizarre example of a 'No-Touch' chiropractic technique was featured on a Seattle, Washington TV station and was preserved for quite a while on the chiropractor's own web site. She demonstrated how she performed what she calls a NUCCA (National Upper Cervical Chiropractic Association) 'procedure' on a woman. They only problem is that she never touched the woman. The clicking sounds appeared to be made by her 'snapping' her fingers.

Anti-medical–Anti-vaccine gurus

Chiropractic has had to reinvent itself hundreds of times over the century. Some of most serious fores have involved vicious attacks on the medical profession, particularly in North America. Since chiropractic tenets have always tended to advance that the body has the 'innate intelligence' (often capitalized) to cure just about anything, there have been anti-medical attacks. Their opposition to vaccine prevention has been raised over the entire history of the profession. But it has really gone over the top in the last decade or so, thanks to the Internet and multimedia extensions of individual promoters.

Professional groups of chiropractors have flooded the market with booklets, tapes, and videos across the world. They often use the likes of holistic health practitioners or self-proclaimed victims to convince whole communities that immunizations are the 'devils work', much like the fundamentalist preachers of old.

In recent years, backed by faulty research by some medical doctors, especially in the UK, they have jumped on the 'mercury in vaccines causes childhood autism'. Communities across the civilized world have been decimated with outbreaks of serious infectious diseases such as rubella, measles, pertussis because of their work. The situation is best exemplified by a single chiropractor's campaign to discourage the use of a meningitis vaccine during a serious outbreak that killed two beautiful young high school teenagers. I was personally involved in an effort to make sure that chiropractors like him would be exposed and brought before their regulatory body. As a result, and after along wait, we were able to force the *College of Chiropractors of Ontario* to create enforcible policies and standards of practice that would heavily fine or remove chiropractors who would advance such nonsense. As far as I know, in no other jurisdiction in the world has any registrar asserted this power.

In the world of anti-vaccine chiropractors who thrive in the marketplace around the world, the Ontario decision has in reality made little impact on their own practices or promotions. A simple search for chiropractic and vaccine on Google demonstrated 280,000 individual hits, and not all of them supported their views. When you tack-on anti-vaccine in this search, there are only 1100 hits. Despite this, chiropractic has not stopped their insane rants against the medical profession. Some recent graduates are game to join the gurus at workshops where they pay hundreds, or perhaps even thousands of dollars to learn how to add anti-vaccine planks to their platform of misinformation that they serve to the masses.

It pays to be a chiropractor — sometimes

Chiropractors in the US have earned the right to bill Medicare, the Veterans Administration, and even work in some military clinics. In Canada, it's a different story. Most Provinces do not cover any payments directly to chiropractors. They are allowed to bill private insurance companies, but not most governments. There has been a concerted move across this country to marginalize payments to them. Despite government changes in many Provinces, they have never been able to reverse this withdrawl of government support.

In the US the insurance coverage by government and private companies has opened up the floodgates to massive fraud. Some of these scams have involved chiropractic pediatric Medicaid bills, and have been exposed on national TV. The bad apples have bilked the system for billions of dollars over the years. The worst offenders have more recently paid a heavy price, and not only been fined, but have been sent to the 'big house' to spend many years helping to straighten out their lives behind bars. Some of these creeps have aligned themselves with crooked medical doctors, lawyers and even the police. Their criminal activities include the creation of fake traffic accidents, or they send in 'runners' to accident sites where they hand out their business cards with the promise of a quick settlement. Private insurance companies, and police authorities across North America have formed a number of anti-fraud agencies that share information across State borders. This has resulted in some back-breaking attacks against these scammers.

Chiropractic strokes and deaths

What is perhaps the most serious problem that has tarnished the image of the chiropractic profession in recent years is perhaps not the insurance scammers, or anti-vaccine fanatics. My interest in the issues of chiropractic associated strokes was brought to a head with the sudden death of Laurie Jean Mathiason, a twenty-year-old woman who died on February 7, 1998. She had 186 manipulations of her neck over a six month period, but her original complaint was lower back pain. Unfortunately, her mother Sharon, despite major efforts across Canada to warn people about the risk of high neck manipulation has been unable to move the chiropractic industry to face the facts. The deaths and strokes have continued despite the risks because the chiropractic lobbyists and professional associations have opposed its regulation.

In Ontario, we've seen our fair share of high-profile cases who have had strokes and some who have died as a direct result of chiropractic high-neck manipulation. Perhaps the most widely discussed case was that of Lana Dale Lewis that resulted in a coroner's inquest that placed the blame right in the laps of the chiropractic community. Unfortunately, nothing seems to have changed much since then. Check on the links in the bibliography for details.

The future of chiropractic

I live in Ontario, Canada where we are terribly under serviced as far as medical doctors are concerned. There are long waiting lists for primary care providers, and of course an even worse situation to see specialists. But, there seems to be a chiropractor on nearly every corner of the city, and their numbers have increased enormously. In some areas of North America, chiropractors may be the only licensed health care provider. They can in some cases peform school sports physicals and provide other drugless medical care to children without any supervision. What they can't do well is to render a real medical diagnosis and provide medical care.

Practices builders are necessary for most new graduates who are facing stiffer competition. Scores of these promoters make their primary living by teaching other chiropractors how to use the system to their advantage, to pad the insurance bills, to keep patients coming back over and over again. They created 'family chiropractic' and recruit newborns and pregnant mothers into their offices.

Some promoters have nefarious reputations and yet they still seem to attract more than their fair share of desperate and hungry young graduates who face over $100,000 in school loans to pay off. These gurus invent their own treatments for the same unproved condition – the invisible 'subluxation.' There are hundreds of individual methods to treat a condition that has never been demonstrated, even by D.D. Palmer himself.

Conclusion—Saving lives and saving money

Despite efforts by some educational institutions to bring scientific training to the forefront, chiropractic has failed to improve. If we did away with all of the chiropractors tomorrow, would the health of humanity change one iota?

If private insurance companies were forced to stop their coverage of chiropractic tomorrow, how many people would be worse off down the line? In my 'biased opinion' as a primary care medical doctor, we are headed in the right direction here in Canada. The government in Ontario has cut off all chiropractic payments, saving hundreds of millions of dollars a year. In other Provinces, there is little or no coverage by taxpayers.

Since the chiropractic profession has never been able to demonstrate that their treatments, real or imagined, have contributed to the bottom line, except for a possible reduction of time and lost wages for low back pain, how can this charade continue without the people taking charge and demanding accountability.

References and Resources

American Chiropractic Association. Coverage of news and general information about the chiropractic profession, and patient-geared health and wellness tips. www.amerchiro.org

Benedetti, P. and McPhail, W. (2003), *Spin Doctors: The Chiropractic Industry Under Examination*, Dundurn Press, Toronto.

British Medical Journal. Response to an editorial by Drs Ernst and Assendelft, as to whether or not chiropractic treatments for short term low back pain actually works. This is a must read for those who would like to hear both sides of the story. *BMJ*, 1998; 317: 160 (18 July).
  www.pubmedcentral.nih.gov/articlerender.fcgi?artid=1114738

Chirobase.com. *Your Skeptical Guide to Chiropractic History, Theories, and Practices.* Operated by Stephen Barrett, MD, and Samuel Homola, DC

Chirolinks. Paul Lee's excellent web site that focuses on the excesses of chiropractors. www.geocities.com/healthbase/chirolinks.html

Chiropractic Economics. The leading magazine, dedicated to practice building. You can find just about anything in their back issues, including links to chiropractic regulators and malpractice insurance companies. www.chiroeco.com

Chirotalk. The Skeptical Chiropractic Discussion Forum — #1 site on the Internet for 'Chiropractic Discussion'. chirotalk.proboards3.com

Chirowatch.com. Dr Terry Polevoy's site covers the full spectrum of chiropractic and focuses on its major problems over the last few years, i.e. Paediatrics, anti-vaccine, strokes, insurance fraud, criminal investigations, etc.

Eric Plasker's Mastering the Chiropractic Lifestyle — another self-promoter adds his efforts to the mix. www.thefamilypractice.net/main/main.php

Homola, S. (1999), *Inside Chiropractic A Patient's Guide*, Prometheus Books, Amherst, NY.

Homola, S. (2002), *The Chiropractor's Self-Help Back and Body Book: Your Complete Guide to Relieving Aches and Pains at Home and on the Job*, Hunter House.

Homola, S., Chiropractic — A Profession Seeking Identity.
   http://csicop.org/si/ *Skeptical Inquirer Magazine* Jan/Feb 2008 issue. An article on chiropractic of major importance.

International Pediatric Chiropractic Association. Promotes the treatment of pregnant mothers, newborn infants with vast array of materials. www.icpa4kids.com.
   See also: www.icpaproducts.com/educational_products.htm

Jailed ex-chiropractor targeted in insurance fraud investigation. He also happens to have been a part of a promotional team known as Practice Mechanix. He ran seminars based on business models taught by the Church of Scientology. www.post-gazette.com/pg/06024/643187.stm

Long, Preston, *The Naked Chiropractor. Insiders Guide to Combating Quackery and Winning the War Against Pain*, Evidence Based Health Services Inc..

Neck911usa.com Watch a startling video produced by Dr Bill Kinsinger, about those who have been victimized after having their necks manipulated by chiropractors. 'Is a Headache Worth Dying For.'

Neck911.com A volunteer group of individuals who provide consultations on complications due to neck manipulation. e-mail: stroke@neck911.com

Network Spinal Analysis Newsletter. Containing anti-medical articles from Donny Epstein's office in Longmont, Colorado. Epstein is associated with WISE.
   www.associationfornetworkcare.com/pdf/newsletters/Newsletter1105.pdf

Park, Robert (2003), http://chronicle.com/free/v49/i21/21b02001.htm
   The Chronicle Review - Journal of Higher Education, January 31, 2003.

Parker College of Chiropractic. Plug into their seminars around the world, and order promotional items. www.parkercc.edu

Pless, Robert and Hibbs, Beth (2002), 'Chiropractic students' attitudes about vaccination: A cause for concern?' in *Canadian Medical Association Journal* (CMAJ), Vol. 166, issue 12. Editorial comments about how even recently

trained Canadian chiropractic students increase their anti-vaccine attitudes as they progress through school.
www.cmaj.ca/cgi/content/full/166/12/1544

Tedd Koren's publications. Koren is the arch enemy of allopathic medicine and has visited Canada to advance his anti-vaccine agenda numerous times. www.korenpublications.com

Wikipedia Chiropractors. An excellent resource that reviews some of the specifics about practices, and its obsolete theories.
en.wikipedia.org/wiki/Chiropractors

World Federation of Chiropractic, Toronto, Canada. Dedicated to the advancement of chiropractic around the world. www.wfc.org

World Institute of Scientology Enterprises (WISE). Helps professionals like chiropractors build their business enterprises.
en.wikipedia.org/wiki/World_Institute_of_Scientology_Enterprises

Michael Baum

Concepts of Holism in Orthodox and Alternative Medicine

Unlike science which is concerned with the general, the repeatable elements in nature; medicine, albeit using science is concerned with the uniqueness of the individual patients. In its concern for the particular and the unique, medicine resembles the arts.

Calman and Downie (1996)

Introduction

The art and science of the practice of medicine have the twin objectives of improving length of life and quality of life. All other outcome measures must be considered surrogates and discounted from this discussion. The objective of this essay is to illustrate how the clinician himself can be an holistic practitioner contributing much to the quality of life, even amongst those patients who are pre-determined to die but also to recognise the limits of his skills and to know when to call upon other agents skilful in the practice of complementary care. At the outset, I want to illustrate my understanding of holistic medicine by recounting the narratives of two wonderful and courageous women that I cared for from the time they were diagnosed with breast cancer. One case presented in the early stage and the second with advanced disease but both provided challenges that exhausted all my knowledge and experience of the disease.

Two examples of the working of holism in the management of patients with breast cancer

I've intentionally chosen the stories of two young women who were pregnant at the time of diagnosis and where the issues of religious faith and the health of the newborn had to be factored into the equation.

Mrs Sarah G. – Twenty-nine years old

This young woman was asymptomatic but presented to my clinic following the detection of a suspicious abnormality on mammographic screening. Fine needle aspiration cytology confirmed the diagnosis of breast cancer. There was no relevant past medical history and she was gravid 1 para 1.There was a significant family medical history. She was of Ashkenasi Jewish origin. Her mother died of breast cancer at the age of thirty-six and her sister was recently diagnosed with bilateral breast cancer at the age of twenty-one. A paternal aunt had breast cancer at the age of thirty-seven.

On clinical examination she was a fit young woman and the only abnormality of note was an area of ill-defined nodularity in the upper outer quadrant of her right breast. Special investigations were reviewed. The mammograms which she had for screening, because of her family history, showed an area of microcalcifications in the upper outer quadrant of the right breast. Fine needle aspiration cytology showed atypical cells but a core cut biopsy showed duct carcinoma insitu and also areas of invasive duct cancer of intermediate grade.

In the interval between diagnosis and the planning of surgery, the patient mentioned that she had missed a period and pregnancy testing was positive.

How should this patient be treated and what should we do about her pregnancy?

The simple stereotype way by which I have presented the case history was intentional. Nothing but the patient's true narrative of her own life experience and fears can do justice to this story. We must recognize that her mother died young and as a result she was brought up by an aunt. We must try to understand what it must feel like to be forced to come to terms with one's mortality at such an early age and the clinical history alone cannot do justice to the strength of feeling of Sarah and her husband about producing a sibling for their little daughter, in other words the pregnancy is very precious.

Next we come to the major ethical issues that are raised by this case. From her family tree and Ashkenasi origins it is highly likely that there is a germline mutation in the BRCA1 or BRCA2 gene. Sarah had already been counselled on this matter, hence her exposure to mammographic screening, yet she had opted not to go forward for the genetic test because at the time there was no proven intervention, if she had tested positive. Now her own cancer has made it even more likely that this extended family has a germline mutation, putting increasing pressure on other female relatives for genetic testing. This leads on to a further consideration of the genotype of the foetus. Would she want to know if it was male or female and abort the female, might it be possible to test for the gene on a cell of the developing foetus if a female and abort the female foetus if the test is positive? Unfortunately our ethical guidelines on these difficult issues are falling far behind the rapid pace of progress at the molecular level.

Next the issue of abortion itself; is this ethical or unethical? Well this of course depends very much on the cultural and religious background of her family. In a largely secular society most patients would consider themselves rational humanists and therefore feel that they should be fully autonomous in this decision. Yet as already described, if the patient was Catholic then abortion would be considered a sin whereas, according to the Jewish faith if the abortion would prolong her life, by even a day then it might be considered an ethical imperative to proceed with the abortion. This immediately brings us back to the issue of epistemology. Although in theory it is plausible that the continuation of the pregnancy may increase the rate of progression of her breast cancer, are there empirical data that support or refute that opinion? In fact the weight of evidence would suggest that, if anything, women with breast cancer who become pregnant have a better outcome than expected, once again illustrating the beauty of the deductive logic whereby a plausible hypothesis is overturned by the accumulation of empirical data. Whilst on the subject of epistemology we then have to consider the evidence for and against different treatment modalities in this case and also be in a position to weigh up the balance between quality of life and length of life, as a result of these different treatments. It so happens we have an enormous weight of evidence that will help Sarah with her decision making process about treatment. We know with confidence that conservative surgery supplemented by radiotherapy will provide the same chance of cure as more radical surgery. We now know that adjuvant systemic chemotherapy in young women with breast cancer, significantly prolongs life but what about the effect of chemotherapy on the foetus. Again it is plausible that chemotherapy may have such an adverse effect on the foetus that in order to provide the patient with the best chance of survival the foetus should be aborted, yet empirical data suggest that once organogenesis is complete, the foetus is remarkably robust and can in fact tolerate chemotherapy. So if the continuation of her pregnancy is not likely to interfere with treatment and thus impair her length of life and if the foetus is tolerant of the treatment, then the only matter left to consider for this precious pregnancy is the possibility of Sarah dying young, leaving a second orphaned child to be brought up by her husband.

This to me, was the most difficult component of managing this case and it comes back to the ethical problems of truth telling. However painful it was for me as a personal physician, I felt that it was my responsibility to inform Sarah and her husband that breast cancer at the age of twenty-nine has a very poor prognosis and whilst supporting their wish to continue with the pregnancy they needed to be aware of the dreadful possibility that the baby would be left without a mother; but then as Sarah reminded me she also grew up without a mother and her life to date has been fulfilled, whilst her husband's response demonstrated a nobility of spirit. He was prepared to shoulder the burden with the compensation that there would always be two sets of eyes to remind him of his beautiful wife. You can easily imagine how that interview ended up with tears all round and even this rough/tough bloodthirsty surgeon had to cover his face with a handkerchief whilst simulating a bout of sneezing.

Finally facing an uncertain future coming to terms with her own mortality, Sarah needed spiritual and psychological support which was certainly beyond my own competence or even that of my nurse counsellor. In addition to her extended family and her Jewish faith we were able to call upon the agency of Chai-Lifeline a volunteer organization set up specifically to work alongside doctors in this difficult and sensitive area.

Two years ago I attended the fifth birthday party of one of my grandchildren. In the midst of the mêlée I spotted Sarah with her cute little ginger haired green-eyed five year old daughter. We exchanged meaningful glances, the only two in the room to fully understand the joy of this moment. Mother, daughter and surgeon were doing pretty well, thank you.

Now to my second case:

Katerina K. – Thirty-one years old

In the quiet doldrums between Christmas and the end of the New Year holiday break in 1995, I was called in to help a young woman make one of the toughest choices that anyone can ever be called upon to decide. In fact, the decision reminded me of 'Sophie's choice' in William Styron's tragic novel of the same name. The young woman in question was a pretty Greek Orthodox girl aged thirty-one.

Four years earlier she had been diagnosed with breast cancer at a time when she was twelve weeks pregnant. The pregnancy was terminated and she underwent a conventional course of treatment that involved surgery, radiotherapy and chemotherapy. She was very keen to start a family and I advised her to wait a year or two. At the time I was called in to give advice, she was twenty-one weeks pregnant and had already felt the quickening of the baby in her womb. Tragically, she had also felt the symptoms of the secondary cancer in her spine. In addition to the severe pain that she experienced, she also described numbness and paresis affecting her left arm. Investigations demonstrated that there were metastases in the spine, compressing the spinal cord and the nerve roots to her left arm. The various therapeutic options we had to consider included surgery for immediate decompression of the spinal cord, radiotherapy to the vertebra and cytotoxic chemotherapy. To do nothing at that stage would have been unthinkable as without treatment she would have become paraplegic in about forty-eight hours. Yet, the most effective treatments to prevent this dreaded complication and to add to the length and quality to her remaining life, would compromise the health or viability of the baby in the womb. Whose life was of greater value and whose decision was it anyway? Was the potential life of the unborn more meaningful than prolonging the life of a young adult?

I was hoping that her own religious beliefs would guide me in this tough decision, but when asked directly she confessed to being a lapsed Christian and asked me for all the facts so that she could make an informed choice. Amongst the difficult truths that I had to convey was the fact that with even the best of all treatments her expectation of life would be unlikely to exceed two years and therefore should she allow a new life into the world the baby would grow up motherless. As an informed and carefully calculated choice she allowed the pregnancy to go to thirty two weeks before delivery through Caesarean section whilst risking permanent damage to her spinal cord. This compromise allowed a new life into the world with an almost one hundred per cent chance of survival in health to adult life. This child is a reminder to her husband of his late wife. This child allowed a beautiful symmetry in her fore-shortened life, denied on the previous occasion at the time of her initial diagnosis. I supported her in this decision from my own ethical standpoint because I was not actively shortening her life for the benefit of the child. This new life started at a disadvantage because of the limited life expectancy of the mother, but the starting point for all works of art are of an infinite variety and what could be a less promising subject than, say, Van Gogh's shoes?

To manage those two cases adequately required a working knowledge at all strata in the hierarchy that provides an holistic model of the human subject: understanding the failure of DNA repair mechanisms in BRCA I mutations at the molecular level all the way up to the understanding of a woman in her central role as mother, wife and member of a faith community.

Using these two cases as illustrations I now want to describe what I consider to be holism.

Holism as a word and a concept

The English language has a rich and beautiful vocabulary. My Oxford English Dictionary weighs several kilograms and occupies a whole shelf on my bookcase. All these wonderful words have precise meanings. The word 'holism' was coined by Jan Smuts in 1926 who used the word to describe the tendency in nature to produce wholes from the ordered grouping of units. The philosopher and author Arthur Koestler developed the idea more fully in his seminal book *Janus: A Summing-Up*, in which he talks about self-regulating open hierarchic order (SOHO).

> Biological holones are self-regulating open systems which display both the autonomous properties of wholes and the dependent properties of parts. This dichotomy is present on every level of every type of hierarchical organisation and is referred to as the Janus Phenomenon.

(*Janus* is the Roman God that looked in both directions at the same time). *Chambers Twentieth Century Dictionary* describes holism in a precise and economical way as follows: 'Complete and self-contained systems from the atom and the cell by evolution to the most complex forms of life and mind.'

Holism in the organisation of organic systems.

To do justice to General Jan Smuts definition of the word holism, we have to start with a 'reductionist' approach to the molecular level, and then from these basic building blocks attempt to reconstruct the complex organism which is the human subject living in harmony within the complex structure of a modern democratic Nation state.

Since Watson and Crick described the structure and function of DNA in 1953, the development of biological holism has grown way beyond anything Jan Smuts might have envisaged. The basic building block of life has to be a sequence of DNA, that codes for a specific protein. These DNA sequences or genes are organised within chromosomes forming the human genome. The chromosomes are packed within the nucleus with an awe-inspiring degree of miniaturisation. The nucleus is a holon looking inwards at the genome and outwards at the cytoplasm of the cell. The cell is a holon that looks inwards at the proteins which guarantee its structure and function contained within its plasma membrane, and at the energy transduction pathways contained within the mitochondria which produce the fuel for life. As a holon, the cell looks outwards at neighbouring cells of a self-similar type which may group together as glandular elements, but the cellular holon also enjoys cross-talk with cells of a different developmental origin communicating by touch through tight junctions, or by the exchange of chemical messages via short-lived paracrine polypeptides. These glandular elements and stromal elements group together as a functioning organ which is holistic in looking inwards at the exquisite functional integrity of itself, and outwards to act in concert with the other organs of the body. This concert is orchestrated at the next level in the holistic hierarchy through the neuro-endocrine/immunological control mediated via the hypothalamic pituitary axis, the thyroid gland, the adrenal gland, the endocrine glands of sexual identity, and the lympho-reticular system that can distinguish self from non-self. Even this notion of self is primitive compared with the next level up the hierarchy where the person exists in a conscious state somewhere within the cerebral cortex, with the mind, the great unexplored frontier, which will be the scientific challenge of doctors in the new millennium.

A modern oncologist is one member of a team. Any self-respecting team these days includes a surgical oncologist, clinical oncologist, medical oncologist, diagnostic radiologist, histopathologist and clinical nurse specialist/counsellor. It is my particular prejudice that the clinical nurse specialist (nurse counsellor) bridges the gap between the clinical scientist and those other disciplines that offer complementary and supportive care. My own team has immediate access to a clinical psychologist, as well as counsellors and I have made attempts in the past to evaluate this service according to scientific principles, with the development and use of psychometric tools (Fallowfield *et al.*, 1987).

Conclusion

Holism in medicine is an open-ended and exquisitely complex understanding of human biology that over time has lead to spectacular improvements in the length and quality of life of patients with cancer. This approach, as illustrated at the start of this essay, encourages us to consider the transcendental as much as the cell and molecular biology of the human organism. An alternative version of holistic medicine that offers claims of miracle cures for cancer by impossible dietary regimens, homeopathy or metaphysical manipulation of non-existent energy fields, are cruel and fraudulent acts that deserve to be criminalized. Such 'alternative' versions of holism are arid and closed belief systems, locked in a time warp, incapable of making progress yet quick to deny progress in the field of scientific medicine.

References

Calman, K. and Downie, R. (1996), 'Why arts courses for medical curricula?', *Lancet*, 347, 1499–1500.

Fallowfield, L.J., Baum, M., Maguire, G.P. (1987), 'Addressing the psychological needs of the conservatively treated breast cancer patient', *Journal of the Royal Society of Medicine*, 80:11, 646-700.

Koestler, A. (1978), *Janus: A Summing Up* (London: Picador).

Peter H. Canter

Vitalism and other Pseudoscience in Alternative Medicine

The retreat from science

Vitalism is the doctrine that life processes arise from, or contain a non-material vital principle and cannot be explained entirely in terms of physical and chemical entities and processes. Vitalism emerged as an important idea in European science at around 1600 but related forms of the belief system have been widespread for much longer than this, have continued to emerge throughout the twentieth century and, no doubt, will continue to do so. Aristotle, regarded by some as the founder of scientific vitalism, believed that the soul was a type of life-energy which keeps the organism alive. Even Descartes, the mechanist, retained the idea that an organism receives direction from a spiritual entity. The notion of a vital energy is evident in the Greco-Roman idea of humours, the yogic concept prana, the Chinese concepts of qi and yin-yang, Bergson's élan vital, Reich's orgone theory and bioenergetic fields, and pervades the pseudoscientific thinking used to explain the mechanism of unproven medical modalities such as homeopathy, acupuncture, spiritual healing, reflexology, crystal therapy, qigong and reiki. The ubiquitous nature of vitalism is perhaps related to its primitive appeal. It has been observed that children as young as six years old employ vitalistic causality as part of their naïve theories of biology.

Vitalism as an attempt at scientific explanation in chemistry emerged from Lemery's seventeenth century classification of compounds as animal, mineral and vegetable. In the eighteenth century

Lavoisier grouped animal and vegetable compounds together and by the beginning of the nineteenth century, fundamental differences were considered to exist between organic and inorganic compounds. The nineteenth century Swedish chemist Berzelius proposed that organic compounds are produced under the influence of a vital force and cannot, therefore, be artificially manufactured. The two types of compound were also considered distinguishable according to how they respond to heat: inorganic compounds can be recovered after heating but organic compounds are irreversibly destroyed by heating. However, in 1828, the German chemist Wohler successfully synthesised the organic compound urea from the inorganic compound ammonium cyanate using the simple expedient of heating and the fundamental distinction between the two classes of compound was discredited. Vitalism has since been regarded as a pseudoscience.

Why then does vitalism continue to pervade the belief systems surrounding unproven therapies? Clearly there is a historical reason. Many therapies have their roots in traditional folk medicines and spiritual practices which pre-date the staggering advances in physics, chemistry and biology of the last two hundred years, advances based upon a mechanistic, reductionist and empirical approach to the generation and testing of hypotheses.[1] Vitalistic rationales for unproven therapies are attractive to sufferers because they offer hope despite the lack of any feasible scientific mechanism and are attractive to practitioners because they provide the gobbledegook for a sales pitch. Although science doesn't support the existence of meridians, qi or any other type of vital force, the more mysterious, ancient, traditional, spiritual and holistic an explanation is, the more powerful and attractive it seems to be. The fact that vitalism is unscientific and posits the existence of an ethereal force beyond the powers of science to detect, may in itself, be attractive to those who can't live with the realities of the material world, are unable to deal with a negative or uncertain diagnosis or prognosis, those who fear science and to those who are unable to understand it.

Is there any empirical evidence that vital forces exist? The answer is no, and how could there ever be? Is there any evidence that vital forces do not exist? The answer is no and how could there ever be?

---

[1] Incidentally, I use these three adjectives with admiration and in full awareness that they are frequently used as insults by New Age thinkers and sociologists who regard modern science as the quaint belief system of middle class males in white coats.

Vitalism generates no testable hypotheses and can neither be proven nor disproven. Detection of a signal on any type of physical apparatus implies that the signal must have a physical origin — it must be a form of thermal, kinetic, electrical, electromagnetic, chemical, gravitational or nuclear energy and, by definition, part of the mechanistic universe outside of which the hypothetical vital force dwells. Equally, even though we can't observe it directly in any way, it may still be there, in the same way that God may be there or in the same way that Russell's teapot may be there.[2] Concepts such as the qi of Chinese traditional medicine are myths which enjoy the same status as religious faiths. Believers cling to the myth despite the evidence, reinterpret the myth to suit the evidence, or lie about the evidence to support the myth.

Even though the existence of qi can neither be proven nor disproven, the related concept of a meridian system and acupoints does generate testable hypotheses regarding the effectiveness of acupuncture. If acupuncture points are specific locations on the body, with agreed coordinates, to which qualified practitioners can reliably navigate, and which are particularly auspicious sites to needle for a particular medical condition, then we can do science. Unfortunately for proponents of acupuncture, the accumulating evidence is that the therapeutic effects generated by needling at the auspicious point, needling at the point auspicious for another indication or needling at a non-acupuncture point are undistinguishable either statistically or clinically in any indication, though each form of needling may be superior to no treatment. This, perhaps unsurprisingly, has led some acupuncturists to argue that the use of non-specific points is no longer a suitable control procedure for use in clinical trials of acupuncture on the grounds that non-specific needling generates some therapeutic effects. For similar reasons, control procedures involving superficial needling of the skin are also being objected to. The logical implication is that we are asked to

---

[2] 'If I were to suggest that between the Earth and Mars there is a china teapot revolving about the sun in an elliptical orbit, nobody would be able to disprove my assertion provided I were careful to add that the teapot is too small to be revealed even by our most powerful telescopes. But if I were to go on to say that, since my assertion cannot be disproved, it is intolerable presumption on the part of human reason to doubt it, I should rightly be thought to be talking nonsense. If, however, the existence of such a teapot were affirmed in ancient books, taught as the sacred truth every Sunday, and instilled into the minds of children at school, hesitation to believe in its existence would become a mark of eccentricity and entitle the doubter to the attentions of the psychiatrist in an enlightened age or of the Inquisitor in an earlier time.' Bertrand Russell, 1952.

accept that sticking needles anywhere in the body is generally therapeutic! At the same time, those selected trials which do show a positive advantage for specific over non-specific acupuncture are still cited as positive evidence for the efficacy of acupuncture regardless of what methodological weaknesses they may have or the weight of evidence from larger and more recent rigorous trials.

What has all this to do with vitalism? The debate about suitable control procedures for acupuncture is illustrative of the process which goes on during the testing of other unproven therapies. When findings are positive, proponents embrace the scientific method and shout loudly about the scientifically proven benefits of their particular modality. When findings are negative or the accumulating body of evidence suggests that earlier positive trials are biased or flawed or simply too small, then it is the science rather than the therapy which comes under criticism. By ruling out non-specific acupuncture as a suitable control procedure, proponents of acupuncture are retreating towards a position where the efficacy of the treatment becomes untestable—as unassailable a position as vitalism, a position which can be thought of as a sort of 'methodological vitalism'. We will have to wait and see in which direction the accumulating evidence from clinical trials using non-penetrating sham needles will fall before acupuncturists decide whether or not they will regard them as a suitable sham control.

A similar, but different process, has occurred in homeopathy. Historically, homeopathy is firmly based in vitalism. Hahnemann believed that life is a spiritual force which directs the body's healing. Somehow, administration of homeopathic remedies stimulates the readjustment of the bodies own vitalistic healing mechanisms. Following the publication of a few clinical trials apparently demonstrating effectiveness of homeopathy, the scientific method was first embraced by homeopaths keen to establish a respectable evidence base for the modality. As negative evidence from clinical trials with stronger methodologies and from recent systematic reviews has accumulated, the science has been criticised in various ways. For example, some homeopaths have argued that homeopathy cannot be tested by randomised clinical trials because the treatment is individualised rather than standardised. When it is pointed out that clinical trials can easily accommodate individualised treatment the reply has been that treatment is disrupted in such trials. This is because the expected responses to treatment, upon which the homeopath bases decisions to adjust the prescription, are not forthcoming in the placebo arm. This is another example of retreat into methodological vitalism (until there are some positive results published). Incidentally if it is true that use of placebos disrupts individualised treatment, then competent homeopaths should be able to quickly detect which of their patients is receiving real treatment and which are receiving placebo treatment, an eminently testable hypothesis. Similar tests of whether homeopaths can reliably distinguish real from placebo treatments based on so called provings in healthy subjects have been conducted but the most rigorous and independent have proved negative.

As well as the 'beyond science' argument in homeopathy there has been a parallel effort to establish a 'super science' explanation of how homeopathy could possibly work based on quantum mechanics. Although I cannot pretend to have a thorough understanding of quantum mechanics myself, I can say with complete confidence that I am yet to meet a homeopath with any understanding of it either. Whether or not quantum mechanics can provide a plausible mechanism for homeopathy is presently as untestable as whether vitalism can, and therein lies its appeal to the homeopathic community. Lengthy and bewildering articles have appeared in complementary medicine journals on topics along the lines of 'quantum field theory as a metaphor for the entanglement process in homeopathic healing encounters', but the authors, who may even be qualified in physics or chemistry, have to admit that it is only a metaphor. It is clear that the laws of quantum mechanics have no known application in daily life or indeed anywhere outside a particle accelerator or the perimeter of a black hole and certainly not at the level of organs, cells, or organic and inorganic molecules where human health could plausibly be affected. Similarly, the claim that homeopathic potentiation somehow alters the 'memory' of water molecules left in the preparation after all molecules have been progressively diluted out of the solution may be a testable one but definite proof that this occurs or detection of a mechanism for how this could impinge on health remains as elusive as that for quantum mechanics or a vital force.

There is an explosion in the number of new pseudoscientific theories which attempt to explain and justify implausible alternative therapies. These include notions such as entanglement theory, biosemiotics, and stuckness-unstuckness which researchers in mainstream medicine have not felt the need to resort to. I contend that they are all modern versions of vitalism which mystify the process through which quack medicine is supposed to work and attempt to move it beyond the legitimate ambit of standard scientific tests of efficacy employed in mainstream medicine.

Even herbal medicine, the most plausible of alternative treatments, has as its core justification an unproven, and difficult to prove myth. If specific compounds in a herbal extract can be identified and isolated, and can be shown to have therapeutic efficacy, why would any rational person choose to continue taking the whole plant extracts with all the associated risks of species misidentification, biological variability, toxicity, partial standardisation, instability of extracts, contamination and adulteration? Whole plant extracts amount to 'dirty drugs'. Yes, it may be too expensive or technically difficult to isolate the biologically active component on a commercial scale but this probably won't continue to be the case with the major advances being made in screening of organic compounds, and in the chemical and biological synthesis of target molecules. Whether manufacturers judge the clinical effect to be sufficiently large to justify such expenditure and effort is another matter altogether. Apart from profitability, which no doubt, is enhanced by the adherence to the relatively 'low-tech' methods employed in extracting and partially standardising whole plant products, the only remaining justification for use of whole plant extracts is synergy — the notion that two or more biologically active components working together, somehow potentiate each other so that the overall therapeutic effect is larger than a simple additive one. The problem is that there is not a single, convincing example of a therapeutic synergistic effect between different components within a single whole plant extract. Careful examination reveals that the examples usually cited all refer to mixtures of different herbs, to preclinical experiments or have not demonstrated that the observed effects are anything more than additive. Furthermore, in order to outweigh the risks associated with using whole plant extracts, it would need to be demonstrated that the beneficial synergistic effect could only be achieved within the context of the whole plant extract and not with a mixture of the isolated components involved in the synergistic relationship. Logically, one would already have achieved the latter in order to prove the synergistic effect in the first place, so when, and if, such effects are proven, the use of whole plant extracts will already be redundant. To convincingly demonstrate a synergistic effect in action, rather than simply an additive one, is difficult and in the meantime, synergy, rather conveniently serves to justify another area of alternative medicine with a very weak evidence base.[3]

Historically, medical herbalism lies at the more mysterious end of the herbal medicine spectrum and in the past at least, was shrouded in vitalistic and naturalistic interpretations of health and healing.[4] Whole plant extracts are preferred because somehow they represent the perfect balance of nature required for holistic treatment of the patient. Like traditional Chinese medicine and Ayurvedic medicine, medical herbalism involves the administration of individualised prescriptions which are mixtures of different whole plant extracts. Modern day medical herbalists, certainly those in the UK, like to emphasise the rigorous medical and botanical training they are required to complete before gaining registered status. They also claim, on the strength of published data from clinical trials of herbal extracts, that medical herbalism is backed by scientific evidence. However, this is an example of alternative therapists misusing scientific data to justify their unproven treatment. The truth is that medical herbalism, understood as the giving of individually prepared mixtures of plant extracts, has no evidence base whatsoever. The evidence which medical herbalists claim as their own relates almost exclusively to efficacy trials of single, standardised herbal extracts. There is no convincing evidence that individualised treatment by medical herbalists is effective in any medical condition. They also overlook the fact that most of the evidence for the efficacy of individual herbs is negative or very flimsy indeed. Even for the most popular and extensively researched herbal extracts such as *Ginkgo biloba* in dementia and *Hypericum perforatum* in depression, the accumulating evidence for a reliable and clinically worthwhile effect falls short of being convincing.

The assertion that unproven therapies cannot be tested using standard scientific methods is widespread on the grounds that the holistic approach to health and the special relationship formed between therapist and patient cannot be allowed for in clinical trial design. This is clearly not the case if testing the specific efficacy of the intervention is of interest. All the non-specific effects surrounding the healing relationship apply in any medical encounter and we

---

[3]   Incidentally, I am informed by an eminent pharmacist that examples of true therapeutic synergy are just as hard to come by in the world of traditional pharmacy (pers comm David Colquhoun).

[4]   Is it coincidental that the rise in popularity of alternative therapies is matched by a general rise in interest by the general adult population in children's fairy stories about hobbits, fairies and wizards?

should do whatever we can to understand and enhance these no matter what the intervention is. If the effectiveness of a therapy depends solely upon non-specific effects, and the therapist knows it, then we are in the field of charlatanism and consciences need to be wrestled with. The 'holistic-special relationship' argument serves as yet another justification for retreating from scientific scrutiny.

An idea related to that of a vital energy flowing around the body is the one that illness involves a disruption to this flow of energy. In illness, the balance of energy is somehow disturbed and interventions such as acupuncture and homeopathy assist the body's own self-healing processes. The implicit assumption is that under ideal conditions, the body is in some state of perfect balance and that chronic conditions, even those frequently associated with ageing can be corrected by restoring the balance. While no one can deny the existence of a multitude of homeostatic mechanisms operating at many different levels in the body, the idea of an overall, ideal, natural balance is a nonsense more akin to the idea of a blueprint arrived at by intelligent design than to what we know about evolution and ageing. Unfortunately, human beings have not evolved to have perfect health; they have evolved so that some of them will be just healthy enough to survive, function, reproduce and pass on some useful instruction to those most closely related to them genetically. Genetic variations and the consequent differences between individuals mean that we cannot all be perfectly adapted to the changing environments in which we and our ancestors have lived. In fact, it is more reasonable to conclude that, because for most of our evolutionary history we were hunter gatherers, it would be highly surprising if any of us were very well adapted to the habitats we presently occupy and the lifestyles we presently lead. The evolutionary process is one in which we have always been out of kilter with the environment, our food supplies, our predators and our parasites. The massive increase in life expectancy brought about by improved nutrition, public health measures and scientific medicine in the developed world is, unfortunately, attended by the consequence that many of us will probably have to live with chronic diseases associated with an age-related decline in physical function, not to mention 'modern diseases' such as asthma, obesity, diabetes, and drug addiction.

New vitalistic, 'super science' and other pseudoscientific theories are being created all the time. The old ones mutate and however fundamentally barmy the treatment is, and however many negative clinical trials are published, someone will always come up with a new idea for how a particular unproven therapy might possibly work and how the clinical trial results are misleading. Sometimes the explanation just involves a long and unlikely string of 'ifs' and 'thens' but also frequently requires some major changes in our scientific understanding of physics, chemistry or biology, a quantum leap in the data or even a 'paradigm shift' of a similar magnitude to that involved in giving up the belief that we live on a flat earth. What ever happened to Occam's razor?[5] When the treatment looks bizarre, the clinical trial evidence is negative and the theory behind the treatment is baloney, then the parsimonious explanation is that the treatment just doesn't work!

Parsimony and ethics in science dictates that our research priorities should focus on plausible and probably effective therapies. However, it is more or less routine that publications describing clinical trials and reviews of alternative therapies, regardless of results or the weight of collected evidence call, in their conclusions, for further research. How refreshing it would be to read 'Clinical trials of zogg therapy have repeatedly failed to provide convincing evidence that it is effective in this or any other condition. We therefore call for the end of research into what is clearly a bogus treatment.' Unfortunately, despite the fact that such calls have recently been made about homeopathy, I see little sign that such a recommendation is about to be followed in any branch of alternative medicine. In fact, the opposite is true. The more negative evidence that accumulates, the harder that enthusiasts try to prove that their particular modality works. It is becoming increasingly fashionable to carry out so called pragmatic clinical trials, which are clinical trials without sham arms to control for placebo effects. Unsurprisingly, such trials are very efficient at generating positive results. It has become even more fashionable to carry out pragmatic, cost-effectiveness studies which have the added cachet of producing a precise and apparently, very meaningful, figure for cost per QALY (Quality of life Adjusted Life Year) using the same methodology as that used by NICE (National Institute for Clinical Excellence). The picture emerging from such studies in the UK is a consistent one — the clinical benefits observed in pragmatic trials are small or negligible; adding the alternative therapy to

[5] Occam's razor states that the explanation of any phenomenon should make as few assumptions as possible, eliminate, those that make no difference in the observable predictions of the hypothesis or theory. When given two equally valid explanations for a phenomenon, one should embrace the less complicated formulation.

standard care costs money, doesn't save it, and cost-effectiveness in terms of cost per QALY appears to compare favourably with the threshold implied by policy decisions about the use of other therapies within the NHS. The problem is that the evidence for a specific effect of the interventions in the indications concerned, something one would want firmly established before proceeding to a pragmatic cost-effectiveness trial, is either absent, mixed or very flimsy. All these studies may well be estimating the cost-effectiveness of placebo and if that is the case, as I strongly suspect it is, then the implication is that any alternative treatment with enough chutzpah to convince patients to enroll in a pragmatic trial, would emerge as cost-effective.[6]

In defence of vitalism, at least it has the merit of being honestly unscientific. We can understand it is a myth and know it is untestable. This is in sharp contrast with the insidious pseudoscientific theories and spurious data proliferating around unproven therapies which serve to hoodwink the dreamers, the gullible and the desperate, not to mention the patients.

---

[6] An irrelevant but amusing example of chutzpah: 'A boy, convicted of murdering both of his parents, begs the judge for leniency on the grounds that he is an orphan.'

Edzard Ernst

Placebo and other Non-specific Effects

An important issue in CAM

Imagine a treatment which, according to the results of rigorous scientific tests, is not different from a placebo. In CAM, there are several such therapies; spiritual healing, Bach-Flower-Remedies, homeopathic medicines, for instance, have all been submitted to multiple clinical trials and the most reliable of those studies do not indicate that they generate effects which differ from those of placebo or sham interventions (Ernst *et al.*, 2006). Now imagine the many patients who have experienced benefit (e.g. relief of pain, anxiety or other symptoms) after using one of these therapies. They would almost certainly insist 'we know it works and we don't need science to tell us otherwise'. In order to understand this contradiction, we need to analyse the therapeutic response in a little more detail.

If a patient or a group of patients receive a medical treatment and subsequently experience symptomatic relief, we (doctors and patients alike) tend to attribute this improvement to the therapy. In other words, we claim that the treatment has caused the change. The main reason for claiming causality is the temporal relationship; the treatment came before the improvement. This type of temporal relationship is, of course, one necessary precondition for establishing causality but it is by no means the only one. Another important precondition would be that there are no other factors which might explain the improvement.

So are there other factors which may have caused a patient to feel better after receiving a medical intervention? The answer usually is 'yes'. Many diseases improve by themselves even if we do not administer any treatment at all. Scientists call this phenomenon 'the natural history of a disease'. In the context of the above scenario (patient feels better after a therapy), it means that the course of the disease might have given the impression that the treatment had helped, while, in reality, it did nothing of the kind. We only need to think of a common cold which takes seven days to be cured with treatment and one week without.

And there are plenty more reasons why even an ineffective treatment could be followed by symptomatic improvement. Regression towards the mean is a statistical phenomenon describing the fact that extremes always tend to normalise. When a patient seeks treatment for a complaint, chances are that, at this point, his symptoms are quite severe. Thus they would, on average, become better over time even if the disease were normally constant. Regression towards the mean can therefore make an ineffective therapy look like an effective one.

Other factors seem more trivial but are potentially equally important. For instance, the patient may have taken other treatments (e.g. an aspirin for pain) without later remembering that he has done so. Or perhaps there was no real improvement at all and the patient only politely said he felt better in order not to upset the therapist. Alternatively, the patient was able to establish a good relationship with his therapist. This in itself may have helped to improve his condition regardless of the treatment he received. In all these cases, the result would be that an ineffective therapy could appear effective.

And then there is, of course, the placebo-effect proper. An inert treatment (i.e. a placebo) can cause symptomatic improvement mainly through two mechanisms. The first is expectation. If patients (and therapists) are convinced that a homeopathic remedy will help, chances are that it does help — even if it is an inert placebo. The second mechanism is called conditioning. It was first demonstrated by Pavlov in dogs. He rang a bell each time he fed these animals and monitored the gastric secretion that occurred with feeding. After a while, he rang the bell but gave no food. The amazing finding was that the gastric secretion started nevertheless. When we consult a therapist, we are in all likelihood conditioned through previous encounters to experience symptomatic relief. Thus we may feel better even if we are given an inert treatment, i.e. a placebo.

So the discrepancy between scientists saying 'this treatment is not better than a placebo' and the patient insisting 'but it helped nevertheless' is only an apparent one. The reason lies partly in the power of the placebo and partly in the fact that a multitude of other factors exist which can cause clinical improvements.

In CAM, these non-specific factors, as they are often called, are of particular importance as the therapeutic success may rely entirely or predominantly on them. One of the earliest placebo-controlled studies of CAM took place at the Mineral Water Hospital (Bath, UK) in 1799. The experiment was conducted by Dr Hawarth to test an invention by Dr Elisha Perkins of Connecticut. Perkins had patented a device consisting of two small pointed rods made from 'secret alloys', one being the colour of brass and the other silver-coloured. When applied to the skin and stroked downwards and outwards, these metallic 'tractors' were supposed to relieve gout, rheumatism, headaches, epilepsy and many other disorders. To test the tractors, Harwarth made two wooden replicas painted in the colours of the original. Subsequently he tried the real tractors and these 'placebos' on five rheumatic patients. Four of the patients experienced symptom relief and said they were 'much benefited' after using the 'placebos'. Then the real 'tractors' were used in the same way. The results were almost identical, 'distinctly proving to what a surprising degree mere fancy deceives the patient'.

The message that emerges is that a therapeutic response (i.e. patient feels better after receiving a medical intervention) is brought about by a complex interplay of a range of factors, most of which are unrelated to the specific effects of a therapy. This complexity has implications which may seem paradoxical if one does not consider the points made above:

- Clinical experience tells us little about cause and effect.

- Patients can improve even after receiving a mildly detrimental therapy.

- We do not need a placebo therapy to benefit from a placebo-effect.

The last point, I think, is crucial when discussing CAM. A popular argument is that 'patients know best'. If they feel better after placebo therapies, they should use them (or even have them on the NHS). It ignores that the factors which can significantly determine the therapeutic response (including the placebo-effect) come as a 'free bonus' with any well-administered medical intervention regardless of whether they are in the usual sense effective or not. In other words, we do not need a placebo-therapy to benefit from a placebo-effect. I would even go one step further: Patients have a right to benefit from both specific effects *and* non-specific effects. Placebos can at best generate non-specific effects, while effective treatments generate both specific and non-specific effects. It follows, I think, that administering treatments which are not demonstrably better than placebos is not in the best interest of the patient.

References

Ernst, E., Pittler, M.H., Wider, B., Boddy, K. (2006), *The Desktop Guide to Complementary and Alternative Medicine*, 2nd edn (Edinburgh: Elsevier Mosby).

Hazel Thornton

Patient Choice

L'embarras des richesses.
The more alternatives, the more difficult the choice.

Abbé d'Allainval (Title of Comedy, 1726)

Introduction: what is choice?

To be offered a choice, on the face of it, is a pleasing thing. To be allowed to exercise our own judgment and free will, and choose—a compliment indeed. It implies the magnanimity of the provider; generosity; their faith, perhaps, in the chooser's ability to bring critical judgment to bear; magnanimity in giving the benefit of the option for the chooser to exercise preferences according to their taste and individual needs; in fact, to respect their desires and their ability to choose. But let us not be gullible. The one who chooses is likely to be at the mercy of the provider. What is there to choose from? If all options offered were equally inadequate or insufficient for purpose, it would be a hollow and unsatisfactory provision of choices. For choice to be meaningful to those being offered choice, surely the range and quality has to be sufficient and adequate to meet all possible choices? Not only ought the choices be sufficient and adequately comprehended, but they all ought also to be unambiguous, properly presented with accurate information, sound and proven suitable for purpose, and accessible. There should be no penalty for rejecting all items on offer.

Ay, there's the rub.

Regulation

Sed quis custodiet ipsos custodes?
[But who is to guard the guards themselves?]

Juvenal (A.D. 60–130)

Who is to determine this? Will there be some overseer or regulator? If there is not, or if the regulator is inadequate, then *caveat emptor*, it must be the buyer's responsibility: let the buyer beware! Let him beware, for example, that there are plenty of marketing stratagems that can be used to manipulate choice — e.g. use of green-coloured bands top and bottom on certain cereal packets have been shown to influence 'healthy' choice. Whether the contents have been proven to live up to that expectation, or whether it should be punishable to manipulate in a consumerist, overly-risk and health conscious society is a moot point, difficult to adjudicate. Maybe it is better than 'Hobson's choice': the choice of the thing offered or nothing — from *Hobson*, a Cambridge horse-keeper, who let out the horse nearest the stable door, or none at all! Unless, of course, that choice is superior to all the other choices! Also, the information about what is on offer can be manipulated by only telling part of the story — the beneficial part. Biased information can be used to persuade, manipulate, coerce, in order to achieve the provider's own ends, which could well differ from the user's. Selective reporting from the best positive results does not serve the customer well. These biases, and others, unfortunately, are prevalent in orthodox and non-orthodox medicine.[1] The buyer or chooser must bring their best critical appraisal skills to bear.

Should those choosing also seek to find out (for their own good) what pressures or regulation the providers of the items of choice might be under; how constrained they might be by regulating authorities; guidelines; peer pressure; or other influences that constrain or influence their freedom to offer, or how they describe what they offer?

Who provides?

We should also consider, will the choice be a free choice — without criticism from the provider, or elsewhere, or will certain choices come with criticism or strings attached? The relationship between the provider and the one who chooses is thus critical, particularly with respect to 'who pays'? As was said in *Punch* in 1846: 'You pays your money and you takes your choice.' But the item chosen may be freely available to all, paid for by some third party or mutually catered for. Or is it a choice that has to be paid for by the chooser, with some of the available choices more expensive than others; or with some perhaps 'free' and others in short supply and expensive?

---

[1] I. Evans, H. Thornton and I. Chalmers, *Testing Treatments: Better Research for Better Healthcare* (British Library, 2006), now available on the James Lind Library website, http://www.jameslindlibrary.org/, without charge, licensed under a Creative Commons Attribution 3.0 Unported Licence.

How is a satisfactory personal choice and distributive justice to be achieved under these circumstances? Whose interests does the provider have at heart — their own (perhaps conflicted, or subject to perverse incentives, financial or otherwise) or their customers'? It can be seen that 'choice' is not at all a straightforward matter.

Relationship of provider to the chooser

Should the chooser have a say on what is available to choose from? If the answer to this question is 'yes', under what circumstances should this be? Choice in a medical shared-decision-making scenario may be particularly fraught, due to the different knowledge bases of the doctor and the patient. Trust then become an essential factor in the dialogue, as does respect for the judgment of the provider, as well as respect by the provider for the preferences and values of the recipient. These aspects of a negotiation do not lend themselves well to regulation.

'Patient' choice — i.e. choice in a 'medical' setting

Perhaps it would be an interesting exercise for me to walk down Colchester High Street today, and consider how much things have changed since the example below of direct-to-patient advertising of two and a half centuries ago. Are the people any less gullible? Certainly their choice is greater, not only between orthodox and non-orthodox medical interventions, and NHS and private, but also in the range of interventions on offer in those two broad but ill-defined now over-lapping categories.

One of the major differences for the people walking down Colchester High Street today is that 'medicine', as it is now practiced, has changed considerably, even in the last decade or so. It is now not necessarily something sought by them from a doctor (either 'free' in the National Health Service (NHS) or privately) when they are ill, but it is a commodity (both 'orthodox' and 'non-orthodox') that is thrust at them in a very well-promoted, competitive market, leading them to the goal of 'health and fitness', with motivations other than the good of the patient in this market-driven society. This objective of achieving a 'Healthy Nation' is promoted by government agencies through public health initiatives suach as screening programmes; by pharmaceutical companies who invent diseases to suit medicines; by the homeopathic industry; by the cosmetic industry; by the fashion industry; by the sports industry; by manufacturers of mechanical devices; by manufacturers of 'self-testing' kits; by health and fitness clubs, farms and clinics. The choice of 'medicines' and interventions today is far greater; the aims are much wider.

This was what was on offer in 1760:

> Doctor Mylock Pheyaro informs the Publick that he has removed from the King's Arms in Colchester to the Crown in Maldon, Essex, where he continues to cure (under the blessing of God) Cancerous Complaints, Fustulas, King's Evil, Ulcers in legs and other extremities, Scurvy breaking out in all part of the Body, Pimples in the Face, St. Anthony's Fire, Scald Heads, Itch, Gout, Rheumatism, and many other Disorders, too tedious to mention. What I have already done at Colchester, Manningtree, Wyvenhoe, Saxmundham, Woodbridge and Hadleigh in Suffolk, since June last, is a sufficient testimony of my ability, and those who need my assistance may, with good effect, through the help of God, apply to their friend and humble servant, Nov. 1760 (Phelps, 1993).

Before this Colcestrian 'Essex Girl' undertakes this survey, I should remind myself of the progression of the profession of Medicine over the last two or three millennia summarized so neatly by Desmond J. Sheridan earlier this year:

> Medicine has never been a static profession. The ancient Greeks took medicine out of the realms of magic and gave it a scientific, ethical, and philosophical foundation, which continued into Roman times, lasting in all for about 500 years. With the death of Galen (199AD) during the decline of the Roman Empire, the curtain came down on medical progress in Europe until the re-awakening of scientific thought almost 1300 years later. Arguably, it was the collapse of the schools of medicine and consequent loss of community intelligence that was most important in this decline. During the past 200 years, the prestige of medicine and doctors has grown steadily, peaking in the latter part of the 20th century. Progress of clinical research during this time based on a two-way interaction between 'bench and bedside' has been remarkable with developments in imaging techniques, molecular biology, genetics, and therapeutics. However, over the past twenty years, medicine – academic medicine in particular – entered a period of uncertainty and decline which has begun at last to cause widespread alarm (Sheridan, 2006).

As Sheridan observes, currently Medicine is certainly not a static profession, and is under siege from a range of threats leading to the decline and uncertainty he mentions. Could part of this decline and uncertainty be because the 'magic' has been taken out of it, so that it is perceived as soul-less and mechanical? 'Bedside-manner' as it was known, is decried and derided: communication skills have replaced it in the curriculum—taught and assessed rather than being prized as an art and an inbuilt skill and instinct stemming from compassion and empathy, and the doctor's vocation to serve the patient, not mammon? Incentives and competing interests were probably less of an issue in former times? 'Bedside manner' is frowned upon now, and has been regulated out of existence.

In mainstream medicine, there is emphasis not only on evidence-based medicine, but also on prophylaxis; keeping healthy; preventive medicine; guiding behavioural change; government public health programmes; opportunistic provision by GPs of advice to smokers, to imbibers of excessive amounts of alcohol and the obese. One hopes that this gratuitous advice is given by doctors who are non-smokers, moderate drinkers and of acceptable body mass index (BMI), (a dubiously useful/useless measurement.) Consent processes in these newer categories are lagging far behind: these interventions should be more evidence-based rather than less, seeing that it is the health-professional who is approaching the patient, rather than the other way round. Better information and evidence for efficacy should be provided in these categories, rather than coercive literature that is offered by screening programmes, for example, if the patient is to be enabled to make an informed choice. How many patients, indeed, stop to consider that they have a right to decline any of these interventions? Offering them with good intentions is insufficient: good intentions are not enough!

However, the opportunity for people to decline to attend for screening, even for screening where evidence from systematic review shows little evidence of benefit and considerable evidence about harms, such as mammographic screening, may be a thing of the past. Political proposals are afoot in Germany for financially penalising those citizens who do not present themselves for various screening modalities, including mammography. Other evidence from a systematic review about the influenza vaccine, shows that inactivated vaccines have little or no effect on the effects measured. There is a gap between policies and evidence with respect to this and other public health programmes being offered. The reviewer states: 'Reasons for the current gap between policy and evidence are unclear, but given the huge resources involved, a re-evaluation should be urgently undertaken' (Jefferson, 2006).

'Patient choice' in the NHS

Researchers who produced the Report (December 2005)[2] of a *Scoping Review* on *Patient Choice and the Organisation and Delivery of Health Services* for the National Co-ordinating Centre for NHS Service Delivery and Organisation R&D (NCCSDO), explained that they felt it was important to include literature on choice made by patients' agents (e.g. by general practitioner (GP) fundholders), because, as they explained 'choice as a market tool may bring contestability into health and other public services to influence providers' behaviour through the mere threat of economic incentives. Choice is also an essential precondition of an effective market.' They found that

- Patient choice of health care is not currently a high priority for NHS patients.

- A perverse incentive structure for both commissioners and providers often operated to prevent greater choice.

- Primary care in the UK has not attracted much interest in terms of choice.

- By contrast there is substantial interest in patients choosing hospitals for an elective surgical procedure where they face a very poor service at their local hospital. (But a Report dated 27 September 2006 stated that a total of eighty per cent of patients in Selby and York Primary Care Trust claimed they were not offered a choice of hospital on referral when the Department of Health questioned them for Choose and Book.)[3]

The researchers concluded that there is not a strong groundswell of opinion asking for choice of provider. They found no empirical evidence about patients adopting or desiring a consumerist approach to health care. Their cautionary conclusion was: 'The key message for policymakers is not to assume that choice will improve quality of care.' Has anyone taken note of that conclusion from that government funded, rigorous scoping exercise?

The Department of Health's stated position is that 'Giving patients more *choice* about how, when and where they receive treatment is one cornerstone of the Government's health strategy.'[4] The DoH produced a strategy paper *Building on the best: Choice, responsiveness and equity in the NHS*. They state that the document sets out how the Gov-

[2]   http://www.sdo.lshtm.ac.uk/sdo802004.html
[3]   www.ehiprimarycare.com/o.cfm?o=7,0,3823,4057,4064
[4]   http://www.dh.gov.uk/PolicyAndGuidance/PatientChoice/fs/en

ernment will make NHS services more responsive to patients, by offering more choice across the spectrum of healthcare. It is a pity that the cornerstone for this edifice was not laid on solid foundations of evidence sought *beforehand*. The King's Fund, the independent commentator on health policy issues, is currently researching and analysing the tactical and theoretical impacts of patient choice.

Choice and increase of inequalities

The Royal College of General Practitioners in its *News in Brief* for 30 April 2006, reported as follows:

> A scoping report by researchers at the University of Manchester and University of Cardiff has warned that there is a 'high risk' that expansion of patient choice in the NHS will increase inequalities in access to care. It recommends that the equity implications of expanding choice for NHS patients are investigated fully, and that steps are taken to enable disadvantaged populations to benefit from choice.[5]

Homeopathy and patient choice

On 1 September 2006, The Medicines for Human Use (National rules for Homeopathic Products) Regulations Statutory Instrument 2006 No. 1952 came into force. Section 1 subsection 1(a) states:

- An application for the grant of a UK marketing authorization for a national homeopathic product is not required to be made in accordance with (a) the second and third indents of Article 8.3(i) of the 2001 Directive, the requirement to submit results of pre-clinical and clinical trials.

Part 3, Evidence of Efficacy, section 6 (c) states:

- The data must consist of at least the results of investigations, commonly known as homeopathic 'provings', which consist of the administration of a substance to a human subject in order to ascertain the symptoms produced by that substance.

The Royal Society responded to this. It said that it

> believes that complementary and alternative medicines, like conventional medicines, should be subject to careful evaluation of their effectiveness and safety. It is important that treatments labelled as complementary and alternative medicines are properly tested and

---

[5] *Patient Choice and the Organisation and Delivery of Health Services: Scoping Review* (Report for NHS Service Delivery and Organisation).
http://www.rcgp.org.uk/patients/patient_centre_home/patient_news/news_archive/pn_april06.aspx

that patients do not receive misleading information about the effectiveness of complementary medicine. Furthermore, NHS provision for complementary and alternative medicines, as for conventional medicines, should be confined to treatments that are supported by adequate diagnosis together with evidence of both effectiveness and safety.[6]

So, *caveat emptor* indeed, if our regulatory agency, the Medicine and Healthcare Products Regulatory Agency has ruled, for the first time in its history, that the regulation of medicines has moved away from being science based and informed by evidence. These regulations undermine the integrity of the licensing regime and the status of evidence. They will prevent and compromise the provision and availability of proper information about healthcare interventions that members of the public need when they are attempting to make well-informed choices in order to arrive at properly informed evidence -based decisions. It makes a mockery of 'informed consent' and is unethical.

It would seem we are reverting to a politically driven provision of medicine, with 'provings' being deemed sufficient for the main regulatory body, and belief being thought to be an adequate basis for provision of public health programmes. Patient choice under those circumstances is fraught with difficulty, appealing slogan though it may sound.

This is Dr Margaret McCartney's eloquent description of patient choice (3 August 2006, personal communication):

> Patient choice: don't you just love it. Like all the bests bits of puffery, it floats ethereally, albeit meaninglessly, yet with such overarching smarminess which ensures that only the misguided or brave dare criticise it. The present Government has made it clear that Patient Choice is what they want and what they wish to ensure that patients shall get. For how on earth could the opposite insinuation be sanctioned — that we should force, dictate to or otherwise command patients into actions against their will.

References

Jefferson, Tom (2006), 'Influenza vaccination: policy versus evidence', *British Medical Journal*, 3333, 912–915 (28 October).

Phelps, Humphrey (1993), *An Essex Christmas* (Alan Sutton Publishing Limited, Stroud, Gloucestershire).

Sheridan, D.H. (2006), 'Reversing the decline of academic medicine in Europe', *Lancet*, 367, 1608–1701.

[6]   http://royalsociety.org/landing.asp?id=5283

Index

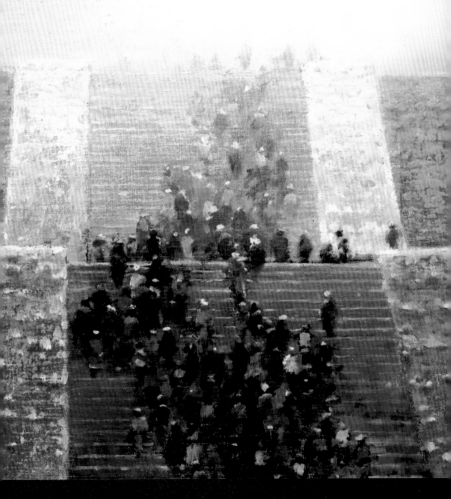

2008–2009

SOCIETAS

essays in political and cultural criticism
imprint-academic.com/societas

Who Holds the Moral High Ground?

Colin J Beckley and Elspeth Waters

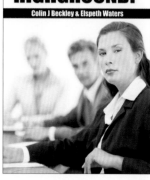

Meta-ethical attempts to define concepts such as 'goodness', 'right and wrong', 'ought' and 'ought not', have proved largely futile, even over-ambitious. Morality, it is argued, should therefore be directed primarily at the reduction of suffering, principally because the latter is more easily recognisable and accords with an objective view and requirements of the human condition. All traditional and contemporary perspectives are without suitable criteria for evaluating moral dilemmas and without such guidance we face the potent threat of sliding to a destructive moral nihilism. This book presents a possible set of defining characteristics for the foundation of moral evaluations, taking into consideration that the female gender may be better disposed to ethical leadership.

128 pp., £8.95/$17.90, 9781845401030 (pbk.), January 2008, *Societas*, Vol.32

Froude Today

John Coleman

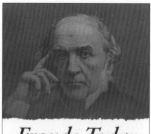

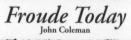

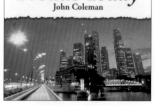

A.L. Rowse called fellow-historian James Anthony Froude the 'last great Victorian awaiting revival'. The question of power is the problem that perplexes every age: in his historical works Froude examined how it applied to the Tudor period, and defended Carlyle against the charge that he held the doctrine that 'Might is Right'.

Froude applied his analysis of power to the political classes of his own time and that is why his writings are just as relevant today. The historian and the prophet look into the inner meaning of events – and that is precisely what Froude did – and so are able to make judgments which apply to ages far beyond their own. The last chapters imagine what Froude would have said had he been here today.

96 pp., £8.95/$17.90, 9781845401047 (pbk.), March 2008, *Societas*, Vol.33

The Enemies of Progress

Austin Williams

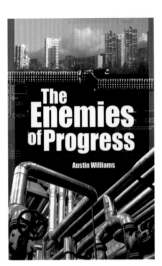

This polemical book examines the concept of sustainability and presents a critical exploration of its all-pervasive influence on society, arguing that sustainability, manifested in several guises, represents a pernicious and corrosive doctrine that has survived primarily because there seems to be no alternative to its canon: in effect, its bi-partisan appeal has depressed critical engagement and neutered politics.

It is a malign philosophy of misanthropy, low aspirations and restraint. This book argues for a destruction of the mantra of sustainability, removing its unthinking status as orthodoxy, and for the reinstatement of the notions of development, progress, experimentation and ambition in its place.

Al Gore insists that the 'debate is over'. Here the auhtor retorts that it is imperative to argue against the moralizing of politics.

Austin Williams tutors at the Royal College of Art and Bartlett **School of Architecture.**

96 pp., £8.95/$17.90, 9781845400989 (pbk.), May 2008, *Societas,* Vol.34

Forgiveness: How Religion Endangers Morality

R.A. Sharpe

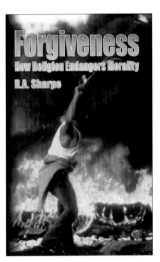

In his book *The Moral Case against Religious Belief* (1997), the author argued that some important virtues cease to be virtues at all when set in a religious context, and that, consequently, a religious life is, in many respects, not a good life to lead. In this sequel, his tone is less generous to believers than hitherto, because 'the intervening decade has brought home to us the terrible results of religious conviction'.

R.A. Sharpe was Professor Emeritus at St David's College, Lampeter. The manuscript of *Forgiveness* was prepared for publication by his widow, the philosopher Lynne Sharpe.

128 pp., £8.95 / $17.90, 9781845400835 (pbk.), July 2008, (*Societas* edition), Vol.35

Healing, Hype or Harm? Scientists Investigate Complementary or Alternative Medicine

Edzard Ernst (ed.)

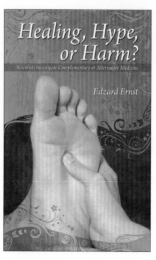

The scientists writing this book are not 'against' complementary or alternative medicine (CAM), but they are very much 'for' evidence-based medicine and single standards. They aim to counter-balance the many uncritical books on CAM and to stimulate intelligent, well-informed public debate.

TOPICS INCLUDE: What is CAM? Why is it so popular? Patient choice; Reclaiming compassion; Teaching CAM at university; Research on CAM; CAM in court; Ethics and CAM; Politics and CAM; Homeopathy in context; Concepts of holism in medicine; Placebo, deceit and CAM; Healing but not curing; CAM and the media.

Edzard Ernst is Professor of Complementary Medicine, Universities of Exeter and Plymouth.

190 pp., £8.95/$17.90, 9781845401184 (pbk.), Sept. 2008, *Societas*, Vol.36

The Balancing Act: National Identity and Sovereignty for Britain in Europe

Atsuko Ichijo

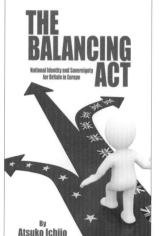

This is a careful examination of the historical formation of Britain and of key moments in its relations with the European powers. The author looks at the governing discourses of politicians, the mass media, and the British people.

The rhetoric of sovereignty among political elites and the population at large is found to conceive of Britain's engagement with Europe as a zero-sum game. A second theme is the power of geographical images – island Britain – in feeding the idea of the British nation as by nature separate and autonomous. It follows that the EU is seen as 'other' and involvement in European decision-making tends to be viewed in terms of threat. This is naive, as nation-states are not autonomous, economically, militarily or politically. Only pooling sovereignty can maximize their national interests.

Atsuko Ichijo is Senior Researcher in European Studies at Kingston University.

150 pp., £8.95/$17.90, 9781845401153 (pbk.), Nov. 2008, *Societas*, Vol.37

Seeking Meaning and Making Sense

John Haldane

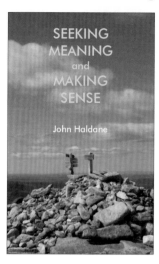

Here is an engaging collection of short essays that range across philosophy, politics, general culture, morality, science, religion and art.

The author contributes regularly to *The Scotsman* and a number of radio programmes. Many of these essays began life in this way, and retain their direct fresh style.

The focus is on questions of Meaning, Value and Understanding. Topics include: Making sense of religion, Making sense of society, Making sense of evil, Making sense of art and science, Making sense of nature.

John Haldane is Professor of Philosophy and Director of the Centre for Ethics, Philosophy and Public Affairs in the University of St Andrews.

128 pp., £8.95/$17.90, 9781845401221 (pbk.), Jan. 2009, *Societas,* Vol.38

Independent: The Rise of the Non-aligned Politician

Richard Berry

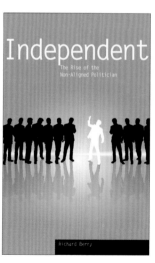

Martin Bell, Ken Livingstone and Richard Taylor (the doctor who became an MP to save his local hospital) are the best known of a growing band of British politicians making their mark outside the traditional party system.

Some (like Livingstone) have emerged from within the old political system that let them down, others (Bell, Taylor) have come into politics from outside in response to a crisis of some kind, often in defence of a perceived threat to their local town or district.

Richard Berry traces this development by case studies and interviews to test the theory that these are not isolated cases, but part of a permanent trend in British politics, a shift away from the party system in favour of independent non-aligned representatives of the people.

Richard Berry is a political and policy researcher and writer.

128 pp., £8.95/$17.90, 9781845401283 (pbk.), March 2009, *Societas,* Vol.39

Progressive Secular Society and other essays relevant to secularism

Tom Rubens

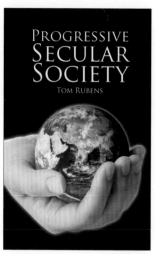

A progressive secular society is one committed to the widening of scientific knowledge and humane feeling. It regards humanity as part of physical nature and opposes any appeal to supernatural agencies or explanations. In particular, human moral perspectives are human creations and the only basis for ethics.

Secular values need re-affirming in the face of the resurgence of aggressive supernatural religious doctrines and practices. This book gives a set of 'secular thoughts for the day' – many only a page or two long – on topics as varied as Shakespeare and Comte, economics, science and social action.

Tom Rubens teaches in the humanities at secondary and tertiary levels.

128 pp., £8.95/$17.90, 9781845401320 (pbk.), May 2009, *Societas,* Vol.40

Self and Society (enlarged second edition)

William Irwin Thompson

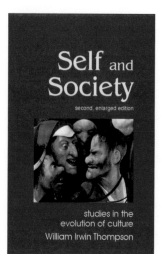

The book contains a series of essays on the evolution of culture, dealing with topics including the city and consciousness, evolution of the afterlife, literary and mathematical archetypes, machine consciousness and the implications of 9/11 and the invasion of Iraq for the development of planetary culture.

This enlarged edition contains an additional new second part, added to include chapters on 'Natural Drift and the Evolution of Culture' and 'The Transition from Nation-State to Noetic Polity' as well as two shorter reflective pieces.

The author is a poet, cultural historian and founder of the Lindisfarne Association. His many books include *Coming into Being: Artifacts and Texts in the Evolution of Consciousness.*

150 pp., £8.95/$17.90, 9781845401337 (pbk.), July 2009, *Societas,* Vol.41

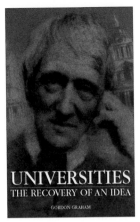

Universities: The Recovery of an Idea (revised second edition)

Gordon Graham

RAE, teaching quality assessment, student course evaluation, modularization – these are all names of innovations in modern British universities. How far do they constitute a significant departure from traditional academic concerns? Using themes from J.H.Newman's *The Idea of a University* as a starting point, this book aims to address these questions.

'It is extraordinary how much Graham has managed to say (and so well) in a short book.' **Alasdair MacIntyre**

£8.95/$17.90, 9781845401276 (pbk), *Societas* V.1

God in Us: A Case for Christian Humanism

Anthony Freeman

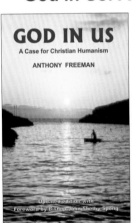

God In Us is a radical representation of the Christian faith for the 21st century. Following the example of the Old Testament prophets and the first-century Christians it overturns received ideas about God. God is not an invisible person 'out there' somewhere, but lives in the human heart and mind as 'the sum of all our values and ideals' guiding and inspiring our lives.

The Revd. Anthony Freeman was dismissed from his parish for publishing this book, but remains a priest in the Church of England.

'Brilliantly lucid.' *Philosophy Now*
'A brave and very well-written book' *The Freethinker*

£8.95/$17.90, 9780907845171 (pbk), *Societas* V.2

The Case Against the Democratic State

Gordon Graham

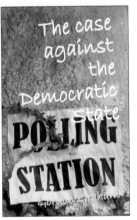

This essay contends that the gross imbalance of power in the modern state is in need of justification and that democracy simply masks this need with the illusion of popular sovereignty. The book points out the emptiness of slogans like 'power to the people', as individual votes do not affect the outcome of elections, but concludes that democracy can contribute to civic education.

'Challenges the reigning orthodoxy'. *Mises Review*

'Political philosophy in the best analytic tradition… scholarly, clear, and it does not require a professional philosopher to understand it' *Philosophy Now*

'An excellent candidate for inclusion on an undergraduate syllabus.' *Independent Review*

£8.95/$17.90, 9780907845386 (pbk), *Societas* V.3

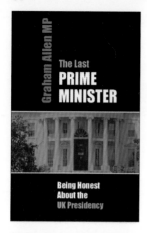

The Last Prime Minister

Graham Allen MP

This book shows how Britain has acquired an executive presidency by stealth. It is the first ever attempt to codify the Prime Minister's powers, many hidden in the mysteries of the royal prerogative. This timely second edition takes in new issues, including Parliament's impotence over Iraq.

'Iconoclastic, stimulating and well-argued.' **Vernon Bogdanor**, *Times Higher Education Supplement*

'Well-informed and truly alarming.' **Peter Hennessy**

'Should be read by anybody interested in the constitution.' **Anthony King**

£8.95/$17.90, 9780907845416 (pbk), *Societas* V.4

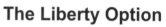

The Liberty Option

Tibor R. Machan

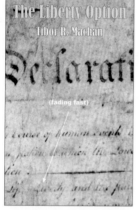

The Liberty Option advances the idea that it is the society organised on classical liberal principles that serves justice best, leads to prosperity and encourages the greatest measure of individual virtue. The book contrasts this Lockean ideal with the various statist alternatives, defends it against its communitarian critics and lays out some of its more significant policy implications. The author teaches ethics at Chapman University. His books on classical liberal theory include *Classical Individualism* (Routledge, 1998).

£8.95/$17.90, 9780907845638 (pbk), *Societas* V.5

Democracy, Fascism & the New World Order

Ivo Mosley

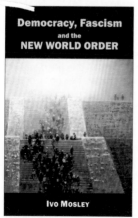

Growing up as the grandson of Sir Oswald, the 1930s blackshirt leader, made Ivo Mosley consider fascism with a deep and acutely personal interest. Whereas conventional wisdom sets up democracy and fascism as opposites, to ancient political theorists democracy had an innate tendency to lead to extreme populist government, and provided unscrupulous demagogues with the ideal opportunity to seize power. In *Democracy, Fascism and the New World Order* Mosley argues that totalitarian regimes may well be the logical outcome of unfettered mass democracy.

'Brings a passionate reasoning to the analysis'. *Daily Mail*

'Read Mosley's, in many ways, excellent book. But read it critically.' **Edward Ingram**, *Philosophy Now*

£8.95/$17.90, 9780907845645 (pbk), *Societas* V.6

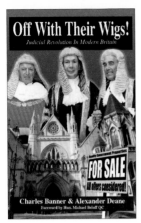

Off With Their Wigs!
Charles Banner and Alexander Deane

On June 12, 2003, a press release concerning a Cabinet reshuffle declared as a footnote that the ancient office of Lord Chancellor was to be abolished and that a new supreme court would replace the House of Lords as the highest appeal court. This book critically analyses the Government's proposals and looks at the various alternative models for appointing judges and for a new court of final appeal.

'A cogently argued critique.' *Commonwealth Lawyer*

£8.95/$17.90, 9780907845843 (pbk), *Societas* V.7

The Modernisation Imperative
Bruce Charlton & Peter Andras

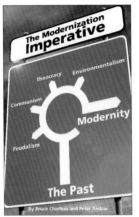

Modernisation gets a bad press in the UK, and is blamed for increasing materialism, moral fragmentation, the dumbing-down of public life, declining educational standards, occupational insecurity and rampant managerialism. But modernisation is preferable to the likely alternative of lapsing back towards a 'medieval' world of static, hierarchical and coercive societies – the many and serious criticisms of modernisation should be seen as specific problems relating to a process that is broadly beneficial for most of the people, most of the time.

'A powerful and new analysis'. **Matt Ridley**

£8.95/$17.90, 9780907845522 (pbk), *Societas* V.8

Self and Society, *William Irwin Thompson*

£8.95/$17.90, 9780907845829 (pbk), *Societas* V.9
now superceded by Vol.41 (see above, p.S6)

The Party's Over
Keith Sutherland

This book questions the role of the party in the post-ideological age and concludes that government ministers should be appointed by headhunters and held to account by a parliament selected by lot.

'Sutherland's model of citizen's juries ought to have much greater appeal to progressive Britain.' *Observer*

'An extremely valuable contribution.' *Tribune*

'A political essay in the best tradition – shrewd, erudite, polemical, partisan, mischievous and highly topical.' *Contemporary Political Theory*

£8.95/$17.90, 9780907845515 (pbk), *Societas* V.10

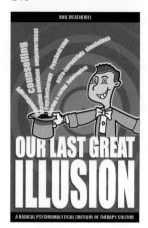

Our Last Great Illusion
Rob Weatherill

This book aims to refute, primarily through the prism of modern psychoanalysis and postmodern theory, the notion of a return to nature, to holism, or to a pre-Cartesian ideal of harmony and integration. Far from helping people, therapy culture's utopian solutions may be a cynical distraction, creating delusions of hope. Yet solutions proliferate in the free market; this is why therapy is our last great illusion. The author is a psychoanalytic psychotherapist and lecturer, Trinity College, Dublin.

'Challenging, but well worth the engagement.' *Network*

£8.95/$17.90, 9780907845959 (pbk), *Societas* V.11

The Snake that Swallowed its Tail
Mark Garnett

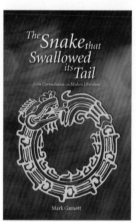

Liberal values are the hallmark of a civilised society, but depend on an optimistic view of the human condition, Stripped of this essential ingredient, liberalism has become a hollow abstraction. Tracing its effects through the media, politics and the public services, the book argues that hollowed-out liberalism has helped to produce our present discontent.

'This arresting account will be read with profit by anyone interested in the role of ideas in politics.'
John Gray, *New Statesman*

'A spirited polemic addressing the malaise of British politics.' **Michael Freeden**, *The European Legacy*

£8.95/$17.90, 9780907845881 (pbk), *Societas* V.12

Why the Mind is Not a Computer
Raymond Tallis

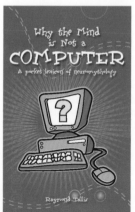

The equation 'Mind = Machine' is false. This pocket lexicon of 'neuromythology' shows why. Taking a series of keywords such as calculation, language, information and memory, Professor Tallis shows how their misuse has a misled a generation. First of all these words were used literally in the description of the human mind. Then computer scientists applied them metaphorically to the workings of machines. And finally the use of the terms was called as evidence of artificial intelligence in machines *and* the computational nature of thought.

'A splendid exception to the helpless specialisation of our age' **Mary Midgley**, *THES*

'A work of radical clarity.' *J. Consciousness Studies*

£8.95/$17.90, 9780907845942 (pbk), *Societas* V.13

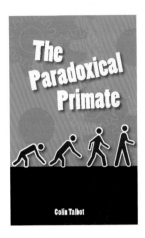

The Paradoxical Primate
Colin Talbot

This book seeks to explain how human beings can be so malleable, yet have an inherited set of instincts. When E.O. Wilson's *Consilience* made a plea for greater integration, it was assumed that the traffic would be from physical to human science. Talbot reverses this assumption and reviews some of the most innovative developments in evolutionary psychology, ethology and behavioural genetics.

'Talbot's ambition is admirable…a framework that can simultaneously encompass individualism and concern for collective wellbeing.' *Public* (The Guardian)

£8.95/$17.90, 9780907845850 (pbk), *Societas* V.14

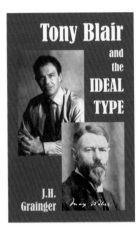

Tony Blair and the Ideal Type
J.H. Grainger

The 'ideal type' is Max Weber's hypothetical leading democratic politician, whom the author finds realized in Tony Blair. He is a politician emerging from no obvious mould, treading no well-beaten path to high office, and having few affinities of tone, character or style with his predecessors. He is the Outsider or Intruder, not belonging to the 'given' of British politics and dedicated to its transformation. (The principles outlined are also applicable. across the parties, in the post-Blair period.) The author was reader in political science at the Australian National University and is the author of *Character and Style in English Politics* (CUP).

'A brilliant essay.' **Simon Jenkins**, *Sunday Times*
'A scintillating case of the higher rudeness.' *Guardian*

£8.95/$17.90, 9781845400248 (pbk), *Societas* V.15

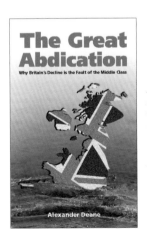

The Great Abdication
Alex Deane

According to Deane, Britain's middle class has abstained from its responsibility to uphold societal values, resulting in the collapse of our society's norms and standards. The middle classes must reinstate themselves as arbiters of morality, be unafraid to judge their fellow men, and follow through with the condemnation that follows when individuals sin against common values.

'[Deane] thinks there is still an element in the population which has traditional middle-class values. Well, maybe.' **George Wedd**, *Contemporary Review*

£8.95/$17.90, 9780907845973 (pbk), *Societas* V.16

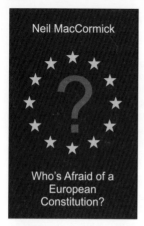

Neil MacCormick

Who's Afraid of a
European
Constitution?

Who's Afraid of a European Constitution?

Neil MacCormick

This book discusses how the EU Constitution was drafted, whether it promised any enhancement of democracy in the EU and whether it implied that the EU is becoming a superstate. The arguments are equally of interest regarding the EU Reform Treaty.

Sir Neil MacCormick is professor of public law at Edinburgh University. He was an MEP and a member of the Convention on the Future of Europe.

£8.95/$17.90, 9781845392 (pbk), *Societas* V.17

Darwinian Conservatism

Larry Arnhart

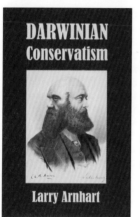

DARWINIAN
Conservatism

Larry Arnhart

The Left has traditionally assumed that human nature is so malleable, so perfectible, that it can be shaped in almost any direction. Conservatives object, arguing that social order arises not from rational planning but from the spontaneous order of instincts and habits. Darwinian biology sustains conservative social thought by showing how the human capacity for spontaneous order arises from social instincts and a moral sense shaped by natural selection. The author is professor of political science at Northern Illinois University.

'Strongly recommended.' *Salisbury Review*
'An excellect book.' **Anthony Flew**, *Right Now!*
'Conservative critics of Darwin ignore Arnhart at their own peril.' *Review of Politics*

96 pp., £8.95/$17.90, 9780907845997 (pbk.), *Societas,* Vol. 18

Doing Less With Less: Making Britain More Secure

Paul Robinson

Doing Less with Less
Making Britain More Secure

Paul Robinson

Notwithstanding the rhetoric of the 'war on terror', the world is now a far safer place. However, armed forces designed for the Cold War encourage global interference through pre-emption and other forms of military interventionism. We would be safer with less. The author, an ex-army officer, is assistant director of the Centre for Security Studies at Hull University.

'Robinson's criticisms need to be answered.'
Tim Garden, *RUSI Journal*
'The arguments in this thesis should be acknowledged by the MOD.' **Major General Patrick Cordingley DSO**

£8.95/$17.90, 9781845400422 (pbk), *Societas* V.19

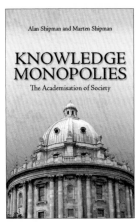

Knowledge Monopolies
Alan Shipman & Marten Shipman

Historians and sociologists chart the *consequences* of the expansion of knowledge; philosophers of science examine the *causes*. This book bridges the gap. The focus is on the paradox whereby, as the general public becomes better educated to live and work with knowledge, the 'academy' increases its intellectual distance, so that the nature of reality becomes more rather than less obscure.

'A deep and searching look at the successes and failures of higher education.' *Commonwealth Lawyer*

'A must read.' *Public* (The Guardian)

£8.95/$17.90, 9781845400286 (pbk), *Societas* V.20

The Referendum Roundabout
Kieron O'Hara

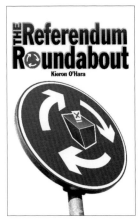

A lively and sharp critique of the role of the referendum in modern British politics. The 1975 vote on Europe is the lens to focus the subject, and the controversy over the referendum on the European constitution is also in the author's sights.

The author is a senior research fellow at the University of Southampton and author of *Plato and the Internet, Trust: From Socrates to Spin* and *After Blair: Conservatism Beyond Thatcher* (2005).

£8.95/$17.90, 9781845400408 (pbk), *Societas* V.21

The Moral Mind
Henry Haslam

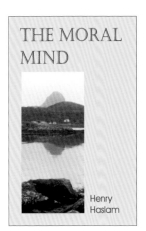

The reality and validity of the moral sense took a battering in the last century. Materialist trends in philosophy, the decline in religious faith, and a loosening of traditional moral constraints added up to a shift in public attitudes, leaving many people aware of a questioning of moral claims and uneasy with a world that has no place for the morality. Haslam shows how important the moral sense is to the human personality and exposes the weakness in much current thinking that suggests otherwise.

'Marking a true advance in the discussion of evolutionary explanations of morality, this book is highly recommended for all collections.'
David Gordon, *Library Journal*

'An extremely sensible little book. It says things that are really rather obvious, but which have somehow got forgotten.' **Mary Midgley**

£8.95/$17.90, 9781845400163 (pbk), *Societas* V.22

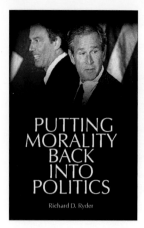

Putting Morality Back Into Politics *Richard D. Ryder*

Ryder argues that the time has come for public policies to be seen to be based upon moral objectives. Politicians should be expected routinely to justify their policies with open moral argument. In Part I, Ryder sketches an overview of contemporary political philosophy as it relates to the moral basis for politics, and Part 2 suggests a way of putting morality back into politics, along with a clearer emphasis upon scientific evidence. Trained as a psychologist, the author has also been a political lobbyist, mostly in relation to animal welfare.

£8.95/$17.90, 9781845400477 (pbk), *Societas* V.23

Village Democracy
John Papworth

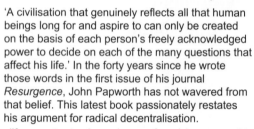

'A civilisation that genuinely reflects all that human beings long for and aspire to can only be created on the basis of each person's freely acknowledged power to decide on each of the many questions that affect his life.' In the forty years since he wrote those words in the first issue of his journal *Resurgence*, John Papworth has not wavered from that belief. This latest book passionately restates his argument for radical decentralisation.

> 'If we are to stand any chance of surviving we need to heed Papworth's call for decentralisation.'
> **Zac Goldsmith**, *The Ecologist*

£8.95/$17.90, 9781845400644 (pbk), *Societas* V.24

Debating Humanism
Dolan Cummings (ed.)

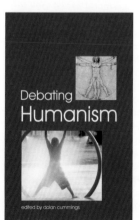

Broadly speaking, the humanist tradition is one in which it is we as human beings who decide for ourselves what is best for us, and are responsible for shaping our own societies. For humanists, then, debate is all the more important, not least at a time when there is discussion about the unexpected return of religion as a political force. This collection of essays follows the Institute of Ideas' inaugural 2005 Battle of Ideas festival. Contributors include Josie Appleton, Simon Blackburn, Robert Brecher, Andrew Copson, Dylan Evans, Revd. Anthony Freeman, Frank Furedi, A.C. Grayling, Dennis Hayes, Elisabeth Lasch-Quinn, Kenan Malik and Daphne Patai.

£8.95/$17.90, 9781845400699 (pbk), *Societas* V.25

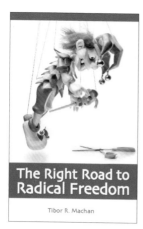

The Right Road to Radical Freedom *Tibor R. Machan*

This work focuses on the topic of free will – do we as individual human beings choose our conduct, at least partly independently, freely? He comes down on the side of libertarians who answer Yes, and scorns the compatibilism of philosophers like Daniel Dennett, who try to rescue some kind of freedom from a physically determined universe. From here he moves on to apply his belief in radical freedom to areas of life such as religion, politics, and morality, tackling subjects as diverse as taxation, private property, justice and the welfare state.

£8.95/$17.90, 9781845400187 (pbk), *Societas* V.26

Paradoxes of Power: Reflections on the Thatcher Interlude
Sir Alfred Sherman

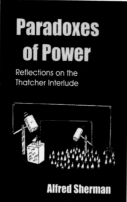

In her memoirs Lady Thatcher herself pays tribute to her former adviser's 'brilliance', the 'force and clarity of his mind', his 'breadth of reading and his skills as a ruthless polemicist'. She credits him with a central role in her achievements. Born in 1919 in London's East End, until 1948 Sherman was a Communist and fought in the Spanish Civil War. But he ended up a free-market crusader.

'These reflections by Thatcherism's inventor are necessary reading.' **John Hoskyns**, *Salisbury Review*

£8.95/$17.90, 9781845400927 (pbk), *Societas* V.27

Public Health & Globalisation
Iain Brassington

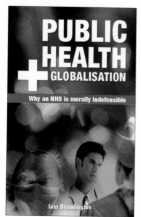

This book claims that the NHS is morally indefensible. There is a good moral case in favour of a *public* health service, but these arguments do not point towards a *national* health service, but to something that looks far more like a *transnational* health service. Drawing on Peter Singer's famous arguments in favour of a duty of rescue, the author argues that the cost of the NHS is unjustifiable. If we accept a duty to save lives when the required sacrifice is small, then we ought also to accept sacrifices in the NHS in favour of foreign aid. This does not imply that the NHS is wrong; just that it is wrong to spend large amounts on one person in Britain when we could save more lives elsewhere.

£8.95/$17.90, 9781845400798 (pbk), *Societas* V.28

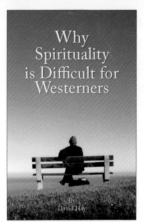

Why Spirituality is Difficult for Westerners *David Hay*

Zoologist David Hay holds that religious or spiritual awareness is biologically natural to the human species and has been selected for in organic evolution because it has survival value. Although naturalistic, this hypothesis is not intended to be reductionist. Indeed, it implies that all people have a spiritual life. This book describes the historical and economic context of European secularism, and considers recent developments in neurophysiology of the brain as it relates to religious experience.

£8.95/$17.90, 9781845400484 (pbk), *Societas* V.29

Earthy Realism: The Meaning of GAIA
Mary Midgley (ed.)

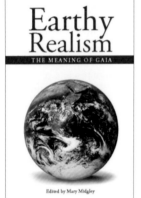

GAIA, named after the ancient Greek mother-goddess, is the notion that the Earth and the life on it form an active, self-maintaining whole. It has a *scientific* side, as shown by the new university departments of earth science which bring biology and geology together to study the continuity of the cycle. It also has a visionary or *spiritual* aspect. What the contributors to this book believe is needed is to bring these two angles together. With global warming now an accepted fact, the lessons of GAIA have never been more relevant and urgent. Foreword by James Lovelock.

£8.95/$17.90, 9781845400804 (pbk), *Societas* V.30

Joseph Conrad Today
Kieron O'Hara

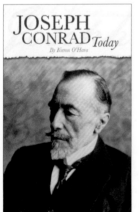

This book argues that the novelist Joseph Conrad's work speaks directly to us in a way that none of his contemporaries can. Conrad's scepticism, pessimism, emphasis on the importance and fragility of community, and the difficulties of escaping our history are important tools for understanding the political world in which we live. He is prepared to face a future where progress is not inevitable, where actions have unintended consequences, and where we cannot know the contexts in which we act. The result can hardly be called a political programme, but Conrad's work is clearly suggestive of a sceptical conservatism of the sort described by the author in his 2005 book *After Blair: Conservatism Beyond Thatcher*.

£8.95/$17.90, 9781845400668 (pbk.), *Societas* V.31